Book Supplement Series to the
Journal of Chinese Philosophy
Editor: Chung-ying Cheng

NEW INTERDISCIPLINARY PERSPECTIVES IN CHINESE PHILOSOPHY

Edited by Karyn L. Lai

Blackwell Publishing, Inc.
350 Main Street
Malden, MA 02148
USA

Blackwell Publishing, Ltd.
9600 Garsington Road
Oxford OX4 2DQ
United Kingdom

Library of Congress Cataloging-in-Publication Data has been applied for.

ISBN-13: 978-1-4051-8551-6
ISBN-10: 1-4051-8551-1
ISSN 0301-8121 (Print)
ISSN 1540-6253 (Online)

Book Supplement Series to the

Journal of Chinese Philosophy

Editor: Chung-ying Cheng

NEW INTERDISCIPLINARY PERSPECTIVES IN CHINESE PHILOSOPHY

Edited by Karyn L. Lai

CHUNG-YING CHENG

PREFACE

This is our second supplement since we initiated the supplement series last year. The first supplement published at the end of 2006 has been a great success. We have focused on important ways of doing Chinese philosophy and have related traditional Chinese philosophy to contemporary issues which are shared by both East and West. In the present supplement, again we come across two major problems in Chinese philosophy. The first is the problem of recognizing the context in which the broad scope and rich diversity in topics and schools in Chinese philosophy have developed, together with their distinctive processes of reasoning and argumentation. The second is the problem of application of Chinese philosophical ideas to disciplines of modern significance such as medicine and environmental ethics. The first problem is important as it relates to establishing a full and holistic view of Chinese philosophy whereas the second problem is directly related to our experiences of life in the modern world.

Now we have selected seven major articles, a number of which were presented at the fourteenth International Conference on Chinese Philosophy in Sydney, Australia. My article "On Human Consciousness in Classical Chinese Philosophy" shows how the questions of major philosophical significance have dynamically developed. It also shows how philosophy is integral to human life in the real world as encountered in human experiences. Tang Yijie's article draws attention to issues of reconstruction of Chinese philosophy through Chinese encounters with European civilization in early periods of modern Chinese history. Nathan Sivin's article is a highly valuable inceptive exploration into Chinese philosophical foundations of Chinese medicine. These foundations have enabled medical arts to develop and become highly relevant for maintaining human health. This in a way shows the deeply set practical interest of Chinese cosmology as well. William Herfel, Dianah Rodrigues, and Yin Gao in their article follow closely the initiative of Sivin in making a more detailed inquiry into the philosophy of Chinese medicine which has not been well attended in the literature. Then we have Karyn Lai's article on the development of interdependent self-person in Chinese philosophy where sensitivity to changes to environment and relationships makes a practical difference. She illustrates some of these ideas with reference to intercultural psychological studies. Lauren Pfister's article marks a strong sense of urgency in studies of environmental ethics in Chinese philosophy. He calls attention to serious lacunae between theory and practice in studies of environmental issues in Chinese philosophical circles today. Finally, we have chosen Antonio Cua's article on *Junzi* to give focus to what a human person is required to do if he/she cares for his/her community and environment.

I wish to thank Dr. Karyn Lai for her enthusiastic effort and good work in organizing this set of articles, some of which go back to the 2005 International Conference of Chinese Philosophy which she directed. I also wish to thank Dr. Linyu Gu for the numerous hours she spent throughout the editorial process of developing this outstanding volume.

Chung-ying Cheng
Editor-in-Chief
Journal of Chinese Philosophy
September 2007

KARYN L. LAI

INTRODUCTION:
NEW INTERDISCIPLINARY PERSPECTIVES IN
CHINESE PHILOSOPHY

The set of articles in this anthology establish the contemporary relevance of Chinese philosophy and emphasize the significance of its insights in an epistemological context that values interdisciplinary knowledge.[1] The articles extend modern scholarship in pushing and challenging traditional disciplinary boundaries. Some of the contributors raise questions that can only be adequately addressed in interdisciplinary research, as for instance, across psychology, politics, ethics, and physiological health. Some others cast doubt on the fields traditionally set out in Western philosophy, for example, between metaphysics, ethics, epistemology, and logic and argumentation. A significant theme that arises collectively from the discussions in these articles is that there were no disciplinary divisions in early Chinese philosophy, of the sorts in Western philosophy and modern Western thought. Hence, a more careful study of early Chinese philosophy could contribute to a more meaningful understanding of the idea of interdisciplinarity.

In "On Human Consciousness in Classical Chinese Philosophy: Developing Onto-Hermeneutics of the Human Person," Chung-ying Cheng develops an original account of human consciousness on the basis of Chinese thought during the Spring and Autumn (772–476 BCE) and Warring States (475–221 BCE) periods. His account of consciousness is explained in terms of three integrated layers. The first is a conceptual awareness of the interconnectedness of entities and beings within a constantly changing cosmos, the second an understanding of oneself as a unique human individual, and the third a consciousness of self as part of political society. Cheng brings together conceptual commitment, ethics and axiology, and political participation in his conception of human consciousness. He considers a difficult issue, the tension between expressions of individuality or creativity and institutional and governmental control. He draws on the Confucian theme of the morally rectified ruler who has a heightened consciousness of the well-being of the people and the importance of their

KARYN L. LAI, Senior Lecturer, School of Philosophy, University of New South Wales. Specialties: early Confucianism and Daoism, Confucian ethics, environmental ethics. E-mail: k.lai@unsw.edu.au

trust. Cheng's argument utilizes a number of themes in Chinese philosophy to make the case for a more transparent and accountable government in China. This is important and timely as there is currently among the Chinese a wave of renewed interest in the indigenous philosophies of China to satisfy their ethical, spiritual, and axiological aspirations. More fundamentally, Cheng's conception of consciousness that is integrated at conceptual, ethical, and political levels may serve as the basis for a profound conception of selfhood. This view of self is important not only within Chinese philosophical studies and comparative philosophy but also in other fields of study.

In "Constructing 'Chinese Philosophy' in Sino-European Cultural Exchange," Tang Yijie examines the development of Chinese philosophy as an independent field of inquiry. He argues that what we call "Chinese philosophy" today is constituted in part by Western philosophy, through the scholarship of intellectuals such as Fung Yu-lan (Feng Youlan) and Hu Shih (Hu Shi) in the early twentieth century. Having been exposed to different streams in Western philosophy, these intellectuals proceeded to explain ideas in Chinese thought in terms of the conceptual frameworks and categories available in Western philosophy. While there are concerns about the potential misshaping of ideas in Chinese thought—and Tang is aware of them—he contends that these developments are on the whole positive. This is because, up until the early modern period, the study of Chinese thought was not clearly distinguished from studies of the classics (*jingxue*), studies of the doctrines of masters (*zixue*), and intellectual history more broadly. Although, in the early period, aspects of Chinese philosophy were interpreted in terms of categories in Western philosophy, the latter also gave form and definition to Chinese philosophy and allowed for comparative studies. Tang urges contemporary scholars now to move on from the modern beginnings of Chinese philosophy to consider its distinctive aspects. He considers a number of methodological issues and constructive strategies in comparative philosophy. These include careful articulation of ideas and translation of terms as well as dialogic interaction between Western and Chinese thought. Tang's analysis accentuates the importance of intellectual history to Chinese philosophy and the dynamic nature of this field of study.

While Tang is cautiously accepting of the influences of Western philosophy on Chinese philosophy, Nathan Sivin suggests that study of early Chinese thought must be more inclusive, and that Chinese philosophers should not artificially restrict their study of Chinese philosophy according to modern disciplinary categories. Sivin, an authority on the philosophy of Chinese science and medicine, points out in "Philosophy and Medicine" that discussions in the *Huangdi Neijing* texts (of the Warring States period—c. 475–221 BCE), which deal with medicine and health, are closely intertwined with other discussions of the same period. Sivin's article highlights the deficiencies of modern scholarship in Chinese philosophy because while it is highly developed in some respects, few Chinese philosophers have also attended to the *Huangdi Neijing*. This is of concern given the integration of ideas on ethics, politics, health, religion, the cosmos, and the natural world in early Chinese philosophy. Sivin encourages the integrated, horizontal study of texts that looks for and understands important connections between ideas in different texts. This also involves reading the texts with an expectation that the ideas therein express facets of real, concrete lives: "ideals, ambitions, frustrations and prejudices." Sivin makes a compelling case for Chinese philosophers to look beyond those texts that are centrally philosophical—the *Analects, Daodejing, Zhuangzi,* and *Mozi*—and, as well, to approach classical texts informed by knowledge from other disciplines including anthropology, sociology, and religious studies.

William Herfel, Dianah Rodrigues, and Yin Gao discuss the Chinese conception of disease and hold it up as a viable paradigm of how illness and health can be understood. In "Chinese Medicine and the Dynamic Conceptions of Health and Disease," the authors seek to dispel mainstream perceptions (in the Western world) that conceptions of health and disease in Chinese medicine are "unscientific," especially as contrasted with Western biomedicine. Their discussion is based on an understanding of the human body as a system that embodies dynamical relationships between the different organs. The breakdown of relationships, that is, lack of harmony between the different organs, constitutes disease. According to this view, health is understood in terms of effective harmonies between all aspects of the human body; it emphasizes resonances between the different organs. This in turn means that continuing maintenance of these relationships is the key to health. The Chinese view of maintenance of health offers a different paradigm of medicine from that in Western biomedicine that focuses overwhelmingly on the state of repair of individual, isolated organs, and on rectifying illnesses with cures. Because it focuses on the harmonizing dynamics of the entire human body, the approach of Chinese medicine may be described as holistic. But this article points out that Chinese medicine is also holistic in another way. It understands the human body as an *open system* whose harmony may be reinforced or disrupted by changes in its surrounding environment. In other words, this view of human health attempts, as far as possible, comprehensively to account for changes in the environment that affect an individual. Here, another important aspect of Chinese medicine emerges: it refrains from standardizing symptoms, diagnoses, or treatments. Clearly, this approach is very different from the classification of disease in Western biomedicine. It seems already apparent from this article that a dialogue between the two paradigms under a conceptual framework that is not already predisposed to one or the other, will expand and enrich our understanding of human health and medicine.

In "Understanding Change: The Interdependent Self in Its Environment," Karyn Lai suggests that there are resources in Chinese philosophy that may be helpful for psychological well-being. From ancient times, the Chinese consciousness of change, its imminence, and propensity to affect an individual, has prompted deliberation about how change can be dealt with both individually and collectively. The awareness of change is incipient in a seminal ninth-century BCE text, the *Yijing* (*Book of Changes*), and is reflected more broadly in the discussions in early philosophical texts such as the Daoist *Zhuangzi* and Confucius' *Analects*. She analyzes passages from these texts to demonstrate that these early Chinese thinkers attended to issues associated with changing situations and circumstances. These issues include, especially, the dynamics of relationships and an individual's place within a larger contextual environment. She suggests that the discussions in these early texts foster and encourage deeper and broader understanding of the vicissitudes of life. Her thesis calls for interdisciplinary research in philosophy and psychology where collaborative investigations at theoretical and empirical levels may confirm the value of Chinese philosophy to human well-being.

Lauren Pfister raises issues about the natural environment and problematizes the lack of enquiry into these questions by scholars who work in traditional Chinese philosophy. Through his meticulous research on existing literature, Pfister in "Environmental Ethics and Some Probing Questions for Traditional Chinese Philosophy" provides implicating evidence for this charge: there is noticeable gap in the literature by Chinese philosophers in the modern and contemporary periods about ethical approaches to technology and the impact of technological advancement on humankind and ecological well-being more generally. This is of particular concern given that traditional Chinese philosophy emphasizes benevolent humanity (Confucianism), is preoccupied with life and nature (Daoism), and articulates anthropocosmic perspectives (Confucianism and neo-Confucianism). Pfister's discussion suggests a lack of foresight or creativity, perhaps, on the part of Chinese philosophers to respond to changing paradigms and needs in the modern world. Indeed, were we to attend to these questions, we might quite possibly discover that Chinese philosophy offers important perspectives on technology that differ significantly from those in Western philosophy, ethics, and science. Literature on Chinese philosophy intimates that there is a wealth of insights to be harnessed in relation to insights on technology and the environment; even a fleeting consideration of the conceptual framework of the *Yijing* alerts us to the integrated nature of the natural world and human life. Pfister's challenge should be taken up especially as the condition of the natural environment is one of the most urgent issues in the world today.

Finally, in "Virtues of *Junzi*," Antonio S. Cua[2] presents a picture of a paradigmatic Confucian individual, the *junzi*. In his description of the *junzi*, he articulates a comprehensive view of the Confucian moral program and how different Confucian virtues come together in this paradigmatic person. Cua revitalizes Confucian ethics by considering how the paradigmatic person might deal with problems in ethical life. His discussion brings out the active aspect of Confucian life, in terms of the *junzi*'s cultivation, embodiment, and realization of virtues. He is mindful of the centrality of historical and cultural tradition in conceptions of ethics and therefore emphasizes the need to engage with ethical issues at both theoretical and practical levels. Cua's analysis is cautious as he admits that his account of Confucian ethics proposes an idealized rather than empirical unity of virtues. In light of actual experiences, some of these virtues, for instance, virtues of character and virtues of intelligence, might come into conflict. He suggests that in order to resolve some of these issues, we need a broader understanding of ethics in light of notions of human well-being and spirituality, society, government, and human good. In this regard, his picture of the *junzi* as a skilled deliberator with principled moral commitments is not simply a dated Confucian ideal; the *junzi* could well be a person in the contemporary world who is morally cultivated and capable of dealing with evolving and new situations.

All of the articles in this anthology share the feature of open inquiry in that their discussions generate more questions than answers. The articles impress on the need for further inquiries in Chinese philosophy especially in engaging with emergent issues of the present, in conference with other disciplines, and in dialogue with other philosophical traditions.

In closing, I would like to thank Professor Chung-ying Cheng, Editor-in-Chief of the *Journal of Chinese Philosophy*, for this special opportunity to coordinate and edit this volume. I would also like to express my gratitude to the contributors to this volume, all of whom have been wonderfully cooperative and generous with their time. Dr. Linyu Gu, Managing Editor of the *Journal of Chinese Philosophy*, has provided warm and invaluable support and guidance from the very inception of this volume.

UNIVERSITY OF NEW SOUTH WALES
Sydney, Australia

ENDNOTES

1. A number of articles in this collection (by Sivin, Lai, Pfister, Cheng) were presented at the International Society for Chinese Philosophy Conference held at the University of New South Wales in Sydney, Australia, in July 2005. The theme of the conference, "Chinese Philosophy and Human Development in the 21st Century," drew attention to the wealth of insights afforded by Chinese philosophy.
2. Professor Antonio S. Cua passed away on March 27, 2007. His article included in this volume, which he sent to me on March 6, 2007, may have been his last completed work. Professor Cua was a deeply loved, admired, and respected teacher and scholar in Chinese philosophy and his outstanding contributions to the field will continue to influence future research for many years to come.

CHUNG-YING CHENG

ON HUMAN CONSCIOUSNESS IN CLASSICAL CHINESE PHILOSOPHY: DEVELOPING ONTO-HERMENEUTICS OF THE HUMAN PERSON

Consciousness is the defining characteristic of human personhood. This consciousness is not simply awareness of one's physical existence but an awareness of one's identity, according to which one relates to and interacts with others, and which gives a unique value to one's existence. In one's conscious self-awareness, one's identity is continually being developed in deepening and expanding processes. In deepening processes, a person acquires conscious self-awareness of him/herself as a unique individual; in the expanding process he/she is involved with others in a co-consciousness of humanity. These two processes are deeply integrated, each informing and shaping the other, through a person's life. On this basis, a human person is embedded in his/her cultural and historical background, against which self-consciousness is formed. The larger social and historical context in part constitutes an individual, but it also inspires him/her and provides a context for his/her creativity. In being a participant of society in its ongoing transformations, the human person, through his/her consciousness, is potentially capable of engaging in the collective transformation of a people in contexts that include ecological, historical, cultural, economic, and political forces.

In this article, I suggest that we understand human consciousness in Chinese philosophy at three integrated levels, each of which requires the other two for both development and understanding. The first layer of human consciousness is a consciousness about the cosmological context within which all life is embedded. This consciousness is informed by pre-conceptions as well as observations of the world. The pre-conceptions and observations come together to form dynamic systems of concepts, and are presented through the symbols and forms of a specific language. Because the cosmological concepts develop from experiences that consist in observation and understanding of the

CHUNG-YING CHENG, Professor, Department of Philosophy, University of Hawaii at Manoa. Editor-in-Chief of *Journal of Chinese Philosophy*. Specialties: Confucianism/Neo-Confucianism, hermeneutics/onto-hermeneutics, metaphysics. E-mail: ccheng@hawaii.edu

cosmic world and incessant processes of change and transformation therein, we may call this system the onto-cosmology of change and transformation of things. In such a system, reality is understood in terms of a comprehensive totality of entities that are generated from a common source, that are interconnected and constantly undergoing transformation.

The second layer is a consciousness of human self, derived from a reflection and understanding of the unique position of the human person in the world, including especially the functions of the human heart-mind (*xin*). At this second level, a human person reflects on his own identity and its defining characteristics, and, in a self-aware manner, conceives of himself as distinct from other people in a culture or in a community. The self-consciousness of the human person becomes the root for moral, ethical, and religious consciousness of human identity; it also provides the potential for realizing one's unique identity.[1] In light of this, we should also consider questions relating to the problems of self-realization especially in regard to structures of social and political institutions that circumscribe and unnaturally repress religious and moral values, whether of the human individual or community. In comparative terms, we should continue to explore how different philosophical systems address questions of human good and development, as well as the makeup of mind and nature.

Finally, there is a layer of sociopolitical consciousness that is related to moral consciousness on one hand and cosmological consciousness on the other. In a sense sociopolitical consciousness represents not only how a human individual acts to develop himself, but also how to relate to others like him so that human values may be realized through a society's institutions and infrastructure. Conceptions of good government in specific cultures and traditions are grounded in their particular cosmological beliefs as well as moral and axiological values. Within these contexts, tensions often arise between sociopolitical structures on the one hand, and moral consciousness on the other, that need to be resolved by philosophical reflection. Ideally, the resolution brings together the highest collective wisdom in a particular tradition. This resolution would reflect not only how a person stands within her sociopolitical society, but also how she relates to her vision of the ultimate reality which embodies her understanding of herself as a human person.

It must be emphasized that while these three layers of consciousness are constructed in theoretical terms in order to facilitate analysis, in reality they are interconnected in terms of mutual implication and reciprocal presupposition. In psychological terms, these layers represent different frameworks of reference and intentionalities, but they are also different dimensions of the same individual. The first layer of consciousness defines the world of being and becoming for the human person. The second layer of consciousness accentuates human personhood based on self-reflection of one's unique place in the life-world of humanity. The third layer is where the human self lives meaningfully in a sociopolitical and practical context within which one can realize his or her desires for creativity and freedom of action. Hence, we may regard the three layers as not separable from each other but as forming an integral part of each other; the actions, behaviors, and speech of a person are meaningful in each of these three layers.

A critical difference between Chinese philosophy and Western (ancient and modern) philosophy centers on the issue of how, where, and when human consciousness on the three layers is formed. In the following discussion, I set out aspects of the Chinese philosophical traditions that express human consciousness at these three levels. This amounts to presenting Chinese philosophy from the point of view of the formation of human consciousness of world-reality, human selfhood, human community, and government. My analysis will cover the period that Karl Jaspers has referred to as the axial or classical age in the Chinese philosophy and Chinese civilization (roughly during 800–200 BCE). It must be remembered that ideals and values developed in such a period not only function as a foundation in terms of which later developments became possible, but also act as a fountainhead for later developments in terms of both innovation and renovation. While the thesis of the three layers of human consciousness constitutes a theoretical structure for understanding Chinese metaphysics, Chinese ethics, and Chinese mind or self, a sense of history of Chinese philosophy can be gained from reviewing some relevant texts in historical order.

First and foremost, Chinese cosmological consciousness is to be found in original texts of *Zhouyi* (also called *Yijing*) which were composed very early in Chinese history. The divinatory practice from Shang Period (1600–600 BCE) relied on texts like the *Zhouyi* for divinatory interpretation and consultation. The symbolic realism one sees in the *Zhouyi* no doubt presents a world of changes that are embodied in symbolic forms of an onto-cosmological consciousness. Later, in the sixth to fifth century BCE, the Daoist text *Daodejing* articulated the development of a cosmogony from reality conceived in terms of void (*wu*). Similarly, the Confucian texts of the *Analects* of Confucius and the *Records of Li* (*Liji*) signify a new awakening of humanity and illustrated a need for the reform of *li* (ritual) at the time. At an earlier time than in the Warring States period (475–221 BCE), the Moists advocated their philosophy of heavenly will (*tianming*) and universal love (*jianai*) as a response to Confucian thought. Following

Confucius, two schools of Confucianism developed significantly: the Zisi-Mencius School and the Zigong-Xunzi School. The texts associated with the key figures, Mencius and Xunzi, as well as the newly discovered Zhu Bamboo Inscriptions, have testified to the forked development of Confucianism.[2] Two chapters of the *Liji*, the *Daxue* (*Great Learning*) and *Zhongyong* (*Doctrine of the Mean*), became especially influential for Neo-Confucianism of the Song-Ming period. It is also necessary to note the ideology of Legalism as the representative of a new consciousness of political reorganization in China.

In light of these developments in intellectual history, one can see how the theoretical structure of consciousness in Chinese philosophy also represents a process of creative development and onto-hermeneutical construction, which is both historically relevant and theoretically significant.

I. REFLECTIVE AND COMPREHENSIVE UNDERSTANDING OF THE WORLD IN THE *YIJING* AND DAOISM

A distinctive feature of the Chinese metaphysical tradition is its understanding of reality as dynamic, and of interconnected events and entities in constant transformation. The central idea in the Chinese philosophical conception of reality is creative change (*yi, shengsheng*) which manifests itself in the generation of life and transformation (*hua*) of states of being and becoming. Change takes place in two modes of becoming, which are referred to as *yin* and *yang*, the invisible and the visible, the formless and the formed, the soft and the firm, the creative and the receptive. Transformation of things in these two modes of becoming expresses itself in terms of growth and decline and in interchange of vital forces (*qi*), which also embodies relevant forms and principles (*li*). Hence, in the real world, any event or entity is both concrete and principled, both phenomenal and noumenal. The phenomenal and the noumenal cannot be separated and their unity is realized in an ontological-cosmological process. The origin and ultimate creative source of the cosmological process is called *taiji*. Based on this understanding, we attend to a number of features of this onto-cosmological consciousness. We understand these features on the basis of comprehensive observation (*guan*)[3] that involves human consciousness across all three layers.

1) Onto-cosmological reality is a source of abundant creativity because the ten thousand things (*wanwu*) are generated from it by way of *yin–yang* interaction. *Yin–yang* interaction can be regarded as self-differentiation and self-integration of the *taiji*. *Taiji*, being the single source of all the diversity of things, is the comprehensive ulti-

mate origin. The processes of the *taiji* are creative and innovative in that they generate all things and bring novelty and new life into being. On the other hand, this process is also one of return to the origin, for all things once flourishing will decline and degenerate and reabsorb into the origin from which all things arise.

2) Onto-cosmological reality is exhibited in the phenomena of heaven and earth. The framework of heaven and earth forms a situational space-time context in which all things occur: All situations embody a history and in turn affect future developments. The development of situations follows patterns of *yin–yang* interaction, difference, conflict, balance, and harmony. The development of the onto-cosmology of the creative change (*yi*) is made explicit in the texts of the *Yizhuan*, which were written as commentaries on the *Zhouyi* by second-generation Confucians during the Warring States period. However, these ideas were already nascent in the ninth century BCE *Zhouyi* text.

3) In the processes of onto-cosmology, the human person in particular is conceived of as embodying a disposition for participation and creativity in cosmic processes. This ability of humankind complements the processes of heaven and earth with its collective development of culture and morality in human society. The thesis of unity of heaven and humanity (*tianren heyi*) is given both realistic and idealistic meanings: A human being is inherently endowed with a capacity for production and creation, like heaven and earth, on higher levels of heart-mind. As a human person is part of this process-reality, he is capable of understanding this process with comprehensive observation (*guan*) of all the things in the world; at the sociopolitical level, he is also capable of contributing to human society and founding a stable political system. Ideally the human person develops and realizes herself through processes that unite thinking and action, like the onto-cosmological processes of natural production and creativity. The human person begins with divination and searches for insights in experience, but she advances to reflective insight into the way of heaven and earth. The ultimate goal of human life is to strive for self-realization in exercising the creativity of *xin*, derived from the onto-cosmological creativity of heaven and earth.[4]

4) The onto-cosmology of *yi* (change) is not theological. Unlike in Greek philosophy where there is emphasis on a transcendent deity or power, reality in the Chinese view arises from an ultimate creative source that is internal to all beings, the *taiji* or the *dao*. The *taiji* or *dao* are also not equivalent to God in Hebraic religion that is personal and spiritual, and absolutely transcendent. In Chinese philosophy, ultimate reality is conceived in terms of a spontaneous process, called the *dao*, with its creative indeterminateness not confined to pre-

determined characteristics. Perhaps it is because of the early presence of this notion of the indeterminate and boundless creativity that no strict personalistic religion has been developed in early Chinese culture. The comprehensiveness of harmonization in heaven and earth also allows a person with these commitments to take all religions as compatible, and to understand them as pictures of human goodness that may be integrated into one's personal belief system. It is also perhaps due to the early presence of this onto-cosmology that there is a lack of mythology in the early history of Chinese consciousness.[5] This is indeed noteworthy because almost all major cultural traditions in the world have a rich repertoire of mythological figures. This lack of mythology in the Chinese thought may be explained as signifying the early development of a rational and yet realistic understanding of natural forces in terms of *yi* and *dao*.

Furthermore, with this cosmological understanding formulated in cosmogony and cosmography of hexagrams one is able to identify things in nature as being embedded in a holistic context of change and transformation, without appeal to localized powers which are often personalized or animalized as mythological figures with magical powers and charms. For the *Yijing* practitioners, nature has its own forms and functions which, through divinatory interpretation, can yield strategies for moral and pragmatic action. As the "Xiang Commentary" of the *Zhouyi* suggests, each situation presents a scenario that requires a moral action to be taken by a human being.

5) Although Chinese onto-cosmological consciousness is not about a personal god, it can be described as divine consciousness in that the "divine" (*shen*) suggests creativity. Creativity may generate what is given from what is not given (or what is from what is not); it may also generate what is not given from what is given (or what is not from what is). To generate what is given from what is not given (or what is from what is not) and yet not to exclude what is not given, or to generate what is not given from what is given (or what is not from what is), yet not to exclude what is given, in the new states of being, links the created to the sources of the creative. It can be, therefore, titled *internal and inclusive transcendence*, which is a continuous transcendence. On the other hand, non-continuous transcendence is external and exclusive in the sense that it creates things from a prior unrelated source and it supervises what is created without being an integral part of it. This form of transcendence is characterized by exclusion and externality and non-continuity.

We must recognize these two forms of creativity in order to appreciate the two models of transcendence as respectively exemplified in mainstream Western theology and ontology, and Chinese onto-cosmology entrenched in Chinese consciousness of the ultimate reality.[6]

6) This leads to the question of creation from the non-being (*wu*) and void (*xu*), which is explicitly developed in the Daoist texts. It must be pointed out that the development of the Daoist cosmo-ontology in the *Daodejing* is not separable from the *Yijing* onto-cosmology. Insofar as the *Yijing* stresses the movement from the internal ontology of creativity to a dynamic and harmonious cosmology of universe, Daoism sees the process of creative change as a comprehensive way of balancing all things and forces and as a process of return to the origin. This process and totality is called the way (the *dao*). Daoism is motivated by a desire to seek peace and tranquility of mind and spirit in the human person, in response to the corruption of human cultures and morality in wars. In this regard, it proposes returning to a starting point where desires and greed in the human person have not yet been provoked and where people can appreciate the natural action in doing no action (*wuwei*). According to this view, natural and spontaneous action embodies a morality which is creative and harmonious for human life. It is in this light that Daoism accentuates the importance of understanding the void. The void is without determinateness of being and is yet full of creativity of being. It is also the formless source from which all things will return. We can see how this notion of the void gives rise to being by non-action or spontaneous action (*ziran*) insofar as being can be seen to arise from spontaneity.[7]

We must of course distinguish this view of non-being giving rise to being from both the concept of *creatio ex nihilo* in Christian theology, and the theory of dependent co-origination (*yuanqi*) from emptiness (*sunyata*) in Buddhist philosophy. The *nihilo* is absolute nothingness and God simply creates everything from this absolute nothingness by his powerful action of creation. The *sunyata* is not absolute nothingness but a state of non-clinging and no-desires in the human mind. The formation of mind is from delusion of mind so that all things we come to know come from a co-origination, which needs to be dissolved in *sunyata*.[8]

7) As compared with these two forms of creation, we must recognize a sense of naturalistic realism in the *Yijing* and Daoism which stresses different aspects of the creativity of a natural reality of which we are a part. Neo-Confucianism in the Song-Ming period combined active and positive naturalism in the *Yijing* with the passive and negative naturalism of *Laozi* in a fully articulated onto-cosmology. We see this especially in Zhou Dunyi's *Taiji Tushuo* (*Discourse on the Diagram of the Taiji*), where it is stated that "There is the ultimate of

nothing and then there is the great ultimate for everything ... the ultimate for everything is also the ultimate of nothing."[9]

8) On the level of ontological and cosmological consciousness, the Chinese philosophers have developed a system of thinking which is radically different from Western scientific materialism which reduces mind to matter. It is also different from Western transcendent dualism which bifurcates the human from the divine and which separates the bodily from the spiritual. In Chinese onto-cosmology there is no reduction but holistic correlation, not dualism but comprehensive organicism. Cosmic consciousness is not separable from human consciousness but exists as a part of it. In cosmic consciousness, there is a sense of origin and the way of development and return, as well as potentiality for creative development from internal creativity that is both transcending and inclusive, both transforming and harmonizing. This naturalistic realism arises as a result of comprehensive experience based on both observation and reflection. Yet, on the other hand, it is also practical and pragmatic because it informs decisions and actions. In the Song-Ming period, this onto-cosmological consciousness was developed into a theory of the harmony of *li* (principle) and *qi* (vital force), which enable one to combine reason and creativity in one's personal and communal life.

II. Individuality and Humanity in Confucian, Daoist, and Moist Morality

With the metaphysical view described previously as a conceptual backdrop, we can begin to explore how discussions of morality in Confucianism and Moism contributed to the development of human consciousness at both the individual and communal levels. We may explain this first in terms of *li* (ritual) as an institution that links human individual development to the development of a society or community, and to the state. *Li* as a system of social rituals originated from religious sacrificial ritual to heaven and earth, and to ancestors of a tribe or clan of people. These rituals fulfilled the purpose of entrenching respect and confirming familial succession. Through them an individual person becomes conscious of other individuals in time and space. The rituals recognize a generative order, a creative continuity, and a functional mutuality.

Li also served to maintain social order as founded on familial relations. In ancient China, these relations were articulated in terms of specific relationships, for instance, between husband and wife, and father and son. The former emphasized respect due to difference and equality while the later stressed reverence due to familial relationship and intergenerational difference. These aspects of relationships became the basis for rules of propriety of attitude, expression, and action. *Li* is hence a particularistic and concrete practice of relating people so that the society becomes not only ordered but also affectively consolidated. In a deeper sense *li* is the sentiment that allows the expression of care for people in concrete and particularistic contexts; it is in this way that *li* is a matter of *ren* (benevolence, humanity, human-heartedness, human goodness). But when *li* is conceived of, or practiced merely as form without the appropriate concern or feeling, it loses its meaning. It is then necessary to retrieve the feeling behind the *li* and this is why Confucius made his call for awakening to *ren*.

What does this *ren* mean? It is the deep feeling of a person that allows him to relate to and identify with other persons. In the ideal scenario, it is a feeling of unity of humanity that is shared by every human being. *Ren* is the consciousness of an underlying bonding between human persons which expresses itself in terms of affection, care, and regard of one for the other. Confucius considered this deep feeling of unity as inherent in human existence and hence declared that "If I desire *ren*, there is *ren*."[10] This means that if one really desires *ren*, one must be aware of oneself as a member of humanity, and seek to exemplify humanity in oneself. This also means that one must overcome one's selfish desires and purely self-regarding interests so that genuine feeling for humanity will reinstate itself in terms of the practice of the *li*. This is the essence of Confucius's answer to the question on *ren*.[11] The practice of *li* based on the feeling of *ren* makes *li* a meaningful and living force that would both regulate oneself "within," and harmonize human relationships "outside," the individual self. It is the fundamental belief of Confucius that, on this basis of order and harmony, rooted in the sentiment of humanity or *ren*, the world will be ordered and the well-being of people secured.

In his articulation of the concept *ren*, Confucius suggests that *li* can be instituted as part of social and community life. With his discovery of *ren*, old forms (of *li*) could be modified and new forms of conduct could be adjusted and made to fit different relationships and situations. In this sense *li* is the rule of applying *ren* to individual relationships in concrete situations. However, we still need a principle of individuation of *ren* in different situations and relationships so that *li* may be devised in these different circumstances. Here, we draw on the individuating principle of *yi* (righteousness/rightness), which enables us to see how different situational and relational elements may be fulfilled by the formation of the concrete rules of *li*. *Yi* and *ren* are related in that *ren* is concretized in *yi*, while *yi* is sustained in *ren*.[12]

Hence we have three sets of relationship in Confucian morality: the relationship between *ren* and *yi* is one of generalization and particularization; the relationship between *ren* practice and *li* is one of a general content and general form; the relationship between *li* and *yi* is one of concrete form and particular content. These three relationships represent a challenge to the old, pre-Confucian order of morality that depended exclusively on the particular forms of *li*. The principles that underlie the Confucian conception of relationships also provide the opportunity for humanity to define its own forms of understanding and conduct. They allow and encourage the renovation of a system of *li*. They enable people to see that *li* is the expression of *yi* rooted in *ren* for relating human persons in different relationships so as to form an integrated unity of levels of relationships. It might be also pointed out that the proper form of expression of *li* and its applications are grounded in the assumption that humans have the ability to see things in right order and to identify an appropriate relationship in a given situation. This power of seeing right and acting right is wisdom (*zhi*) which needs to be refined by practice and experience. A person who attains *zhi* will not be perplexed, just as a person who attains *ren* will not be anxious. This is because a person with *ren* becomes his true self, while a person with *zhi* knows how to apply himself or to discover or formulate the right form of action and right rule of conduct. Confucius also speaks of moral courage (*yong*) as absence of fear. When one acts in a sprit of *yi*, rightness, with the genuine heart of *ren*, there is a natural absence of fear, and there is moral courage.

Confucius takes *ren* as the basis of both personal morality and ethical behavior in society. If by ethics we mean those social norms that govern human relationships, it is clear that they are grounded in *ren*. The ethical meaning of *ren* inevitably points to practice of *li* (propriety) and *yi* (righteousness) which could be said to form the essence of communal harmony, and good government. It is clear that in order to achieve a good government that administers righteousness (*yi*), both *ren* and *zhi* are critical, as we shall see. One dimension of *ren* refers to the deep bond of universal humanity with heaven, conceived as the ultimate metaphysical source of humanity. It is here, with reference to this ultimate source of humanity, that we find the *dao* of Confucius. In this sense of the *dao*, Confucius says that if one hears the *dao* in the morning, one could die in the evening.[13] This is because the *dao* when embodied fulfills the individual and enables her to be aware of her potential creativity in relation to ultimate reality.

We may see this uplifting aspect of *ren* in terms of how it deepens and heightens the sense of self. This is to be contrasted with the horizontal and expanding sense of *ren* which finds itself in the encirclement of family, clan, community, and ultimately the entire human population. We can see *ren* in either of these ways as a form of transcendence, a transcendence of inclusion and absorption as earlier described. In the ideal state the vertical uplifting sense of *ren* could even include the horizontal and expanding sense of *ren* (while the latter may not include the former), and it is in this ideal state that we can see how moral consciousness in Confucianism comes to a full realization of humanity in a person.

Hence, *ren* may function in a way similar to practical reason in Kant's moral philosophy, and which gives rise to universal and necessary principles of human conduct. It also reveals the onto-cosmological depth in Confucius's view of life that is also spiritual in a profound sense. Here, as a human person, I should commit myself to the realization of *ren* as a principle of life and consequently I should practice love and care for humanity at any time and anywhere. In practicing *ren* one will become truly righteous and truly wise. One would thus come to an experience and embodiment of ultimate reality in the activities of participating in the creative transformation of people and things in the world.

In his conception of *ren*, Confucius has inspired a robust development of Confucianism in *Mencius* and *Zhongyong* on the one hand, and *Daxue* and *Xunzi* on the other. For Mencius, it is this experience and vision of *ren* which leads him to posit that the innate nature of the human person gives rise to four fundamental feelings of morality, that is, sympathetic care, self-restraint, reverence, and distinction between right and wrong. The importance of recognizing an innate moral nature as source of morality is a significant move because it explicitly defines the essence of human being as a moral being. For *Zhongyong*, again, human nature is explicitly recognized as derived from heaven or the mandate of heaven (*tianming*) and hence is capable of participating in the creative and ceaseless creation and preservation of being. In addition to this, *Zhongyong* further identifies *ren* in terms of sincerity, that is, by having a complete reflection of oneself without self-deception and without withholding oneself from reality, one's mind will be illuminated. To be illuminated in mind is to see reality as not separate from oneself; this enables a person to reinforce his or her openness and sincerity so that a more inclusive and deepened experience of reality is possible. In the language of the *Zhongyong*, a human person attains realization in his co-creative production and nurturing of things together with heaven and earth, exhibiting a unity of triad of the ultimate reality.

The *Mencius* and *Zhongyong* have emphatically expounded on the upward-transcending aspect of Confucian *ren* (or *ren* in a vertical uplifting sense). By contrast, the *Daxue* and *Xunzi* can be seen to present the widening-transcending aspect of Confucian *ren* (or *ren* in a horizontal expanding sense). In the *Daxue*, a person starts with the investigation of things and extension of knowledge in order to realize one's nature. This broadening process is one that instills order and harmony in family, state, and the world. Unlike the *Zhongyong* that relates the self to ultimate reality, *Daxue* confronts the self with the extended world of things so that the self has to have an experiential understanding of the real world before it can relate to things and then to other people. Zhuxi (1130–1200) later interprets this understanding of things in terms of the knowledge of the principles that would illuminate things.

It is interesting to see that in the *Daxue*, sincere intention (*chengyi*) is based on correct understanding of the world of things and hence is geared toward correct action in the world that would in the final analysis generate unity and goodness. In extending one's relations, it is necessary to see that one should act right and this means to act in accordance with the principle of reciprocity (*jiejuzhidao*). This principle of reciprocity is an application of the *ren* as a principle, which is first formulated in the *Analects* in terms of the requirement that one should not do to others what one would not want others to do to oneself. It is through such a principle of interpersonal practicality that *ren* feeling can be implemented. The ultimate goal of *Daxue* as announced in the beginning of the text is to illuminate bright virtue (*mingde*) and to revitalize and love people before reaching supreme goodness. It is apparent that supreme goodness is the great peace to be established among all nations and all peoples. This is an ambitious task, but it also sets up a desirable ideal of extending one's relationships in order to attain peace in the human world. It is on this basis that the "Liyun" chapter of the *Liji* speaks of the Great Unity (*datong*) of the world in which universal peace and universal well-being will be established.

As Xunzi holds that human nature to all appearances is selfish, he seems to contradict Mencius who takes human nature as innately good. However, there exists no real contradiction between the two. We may understand Mencius as speaking of a deep human nature with moral sentiments, and Xunzi as speaking of an instinctive physical nature dominated by selfish desires and self-interests. We can reconcile both by thinking of human nature in terms of two integrated levels, the moral and the physical. This seems to be a more adequate image of the human person. While Mencius recognizes our physical nature besides our moral nature, Xunzi recognizes a rational human mind, which, when divested of desires and prejudices, reveals a state of great purity and clarity (*daqingming*) that seems to be equivalent to *Daxue*'s notion of "bright virtue."[14] However, there may be one crucial difference, and that is that whereas the bright virtue of *Daxue* focuses on one's ability to love and revitalize people on the basis of

one's self-cultivation and cultivation of moral relations, the *daqingming* of Xunzi focuses on renovating people with institutional design
for education and governmental organization.

What is to be carefully distinguished in Xunzi is that he expects the
sage to perform the role of organizing and ruling people with systems
of *li*. In other words, Xunzi's approach to renovation of the people is
primarily political and economical rather than moral. His arguments
also reflect a rational and even rationalistic concern and understanding of the social and political issues in the community beyond familial
boundaries. He believed that it is only through rational reflection and
empirical learning, and finally institutional planning, that a well-
ordered state and a peaceful world can be attained. In this sense, he
has advanced beyond what Confucius has said about ruling a state by
ren; what he has done is to indicate that *ren* without reason or *li*
(principle) cannot make its full impact. Confucian *zhi*, wisdom, needs
to be developed so that political transformation toward a society of *li*
(ritual) would become a reality.

It is obvious that classical Confucianism has developed a view of
morality that integrates humanities, education, and even religious
well-being. It has a comprehensive coverage that includes moral,
religious, social, and political consciousness. Furthermore, the unity
among these aspects makes Confucian philosophy a unique system
based not on a single idea or value, but on a unity of principles and
ideas of *ren* and *li*. This system is truly both knowledge and value,
integrating both the theoretical and the practical. As this system is
continuous and co-terminous with the onto-cosmology described in
the first section, it can be regarded as a human expression of the
onto-cosmology which leads to the unity of heaven and the human
(*tianren heyi*) through a unified process of self-reflection, self-
cultivation, and self-practice (*zhixing heyi*).

At this point, we need to note two alternative systems that exhibit
equivalent consciousness of totality and human action. Both systems
are critical of the Confucian system: Daoism rejects the practice of *li*,
and more fundamentally, the invention and development of culture
and knowledge. Daoism advocates a spontaneous reality that is free
from fragmentation and strife, and of human invention and artifice.
We see here a critical consciousness of natural understanding which
values non-action and naturalness. This no doubt provides an important resource for the re-evaluation of human morality and human
action.

There are two great classical Daoist figures who respectively represent the initiation and development of philosophical Daoism: Laozi
and Zhuangzi. Laozi presents the *dao* as a source of being from which
things rise and to which they would return. He urges a simple style of

living that is consistent with the primordial *dao*. His vision of reality is in fact a partial adaptation from the *Yijing*'s onto-cosmology with an emphasis on the principle of receptivity and passivity as the ground and as reason for the natural creation of the world, and hence as the model for human life. In this light, he sees human culture as blocking the *dao*. For Zhuangzi, however, the emphasis is on how one may practice the non-separation between oneself and *dao* where *dao* is embodied in all things in the world. The whole world of being is to be understood by an open and creative mind that is not constricted by conventional human values.

Second, Moist philosophy as represented by Mozi criticizes Confucianism also for its excessive engagement with *li* and thus for its lack of universality and productivity. In the spirit of *li* (ritual and propriety) the Confucians practice *ren* as self-control and graded love that Mozi sees as leading to a society of hierarchy of difference and circles of dissension. Mozi diagnoses the cause of continuous wars as the lack of concern among people. He advocates the doctrine of universal love (*jianai*) as the method to attain peace. Love is universal (*jian*) if it can be shared on an equal basis. Thus, one should love other people's family as one loves one's own family. The gist of Mozi's concern is that we should not love our own family to the exclusion of other families in consideration of benefits to be shared. (But later Mencius misinterprets this to mean treating another person's father as my own father and thus denying the unique status of one's own father.) The doctrine of universal love if universally practiced would eliminate wars because it allows each group of people or state to care for its own land and property without trying to ravage lands of other states and other groups of people. There is also the more desirable consequence of this doctrine, namely, the mutual benefiting among states and peoples. This leads to the ultimate ideal of Mozi: Every person and every state would live on an equitable basis and human society would flourish just as a natural society might flourish under the compassionate will of heaven.

Mozi sees the continuous wars at his time as an inevitable result of an inequitable society that lacks a sense of social justice. What then is social justice? According to Mozi, social justice must be founded on one identical standard so that there would be no disagreement on what social justice is. He uses the same term "*yi*" Confucius used, but with an objective meaning. To establish his concept *yi*, Mozi appeals to the will of heaven (*tianzhi*) with which everyone should comply. He regards the will of heaven as the standard of the *yi*. Nevertheless, his doctrine of identity compliance (*shangtong*) is hierarchical as the common people are to subscribe to the hierarchy of ranks that enforce compliance. This would amount to enforcing the ideology of leaders, who may well have totalitarian aims, in the name of the *tianzhi*.

The social idealism of Mozi is criticized for its unrealistic and utopian projections. But a more serious difficulty is the contradiction between his prescription for social justice on the basis of identification with one's superiors and his argument for equitable love of mutual benefit. He loses sight of the individuality of each person and each human relationship. The problem results from his lack of consideration of the feelings and moral freedom of the individuals, which the Confucians make great efforts to evince, and which is for them the natural basis of society and government.

III. Axiology and Political Consciousness in Confucianism as the Mainstream Philosophy

I have discussed onto-cosmological understanding in Chinese philosophy as the first layer of the human consciousness. This was followed by a development of ideas pertaining to human individuality and humanity in Confucian philosophy, which is the core of the second layer of the human consciousness under discussion. It is necessary to note that consciousness of the human self cannot be fully comprehended without reference to an underlying onto-cosmology that is developed in the *Yizhuan* Commentaries of the *Yijing*. Confucian philosophy of humanity as practical care for all human beings in light of their common roots and common ends likewise cannot be understood apart from this onto-cosmology. It is on the basis of this understanding that the Confucian idea of the human individual is relational, virtue-based, and holistically oriented. Yet the Confucian self is an entity that has its own individuality and integrative unity which consciously participates with heaven in its ideal state.

This Confucian position contrasts with Daoist and Moist views of human consciousness. In the case of Daoism, the distrust of the culture of *ren* and *li* leads to a pristine naturalism that is nevertheless consistent with the onto-cosmology of the *Yi*. On the other hand, in the case of Moism, the desire to resolve unjust wars at the time led the Moists to rational reflection and a search for a program to implement social justice and to attain an equitable economy from productive work. But Mozi's rational reflection is not thorough and consistent as it is blind to the rich content of human nature. In this sense, it represents an incomplete and often confused state of consciousness of rationality, which in a later development received more precise and sophisticated definition in Later Moist thought. In the Later Moists' texts we find fundamental terms of Moist doctrine such as identity (*tong*), difference (*yi*), reasons (*gu*), and inferences (*tui*) logically defined and explained. This is no doubt a great achievement insofar as logical, analytical, and abstract rational consciousness in Chinese philosophy is concerned. Unfortunately, this line of thought did not continue and was set to remain in a germinal state in the Classical Period in Chinese philosophy until rediscovered in the modern era.

Since Daoist and the Moist philosophy did not become the guiding principles for political governance in Chinese history after the Warring States period (481–221 BCE), we may ask why Confucianism became the dominant political ideology in the early Han and hence the mainstream moral and political axiology in Han and post-Qin Chinese history. In order to answer this question, we have to understand how the Legalist School (*fajia*) and legalist politics also failed in the period of Qin (221–206 BCE) that preceded the Han (206 BCE–220 CE). Legalism was represented by a trend of thought focusing on the waging of administrative power and punitive laws and regulations that culminated in Han Fei's philosophy. It is a system of ideas which promotes and argues for intentional employment of the political power in both objective institutions and personal orders of the ruler for the purpose of strict control and domination. In this sense the notion of law (*fa*) as a tool of punishment is too narrow a representation of the use of law but is used in such a way to the exclusion and at the expense of morality. It is based on a manipulation of human psychology, of people's desire for reward and fear of punishment, with total disregard for human needs of freedom and trust. Because of this narrow application of the law, Legalism became identified with strict authoritarianism during the Qin rulership, which is couched in laws and regulations driven by the ruler's desire for his own power and wealth. Its failure to address equally fundamental and important needs in human nature dooms the Qin power to a short span despite its great work in unifying China. It also laid the foundation for a need and desire to return to Confucianism as a humanistic moral tradition.

The return to Confucianism and especially to its political consciousness in the early Han is in many ways an outcome necessitated by the historical circumstances after the collapse of the Qin in the third century BCE. In fact, to choose to embrace Confucianism as its state ideology is a natural and reasonable choice for the Han Emperor Wudi because there were no better alternatives as far as political governance was concerned. Confucianism presented an axiology of integrated values which have historical roots and which could be redefined in political terms to regulate the behavior of the people. The Confucian axiology of values I am speaking of here are the Confucian virtues which reflect a concept of malleable human nature capable of achieving a unification of the inner moral consciousness with the outer cosmic consciousness.

This is precisely the central tenet of Dong Zhongshu (179–104 BCE) who developed Confucian political ideology that legitimized political rule. Dong speaks of harmonization and preservation of humanity and community as the primary concern of a ruler who should extend his *ren* from the moral domain to the domain of political control. Thus, he is able to transform the values of five virtuous relationships into three basic norms of organization and leadership: The people obey the ruler, the son obeys the father, and the wife obeys the husband.[15] This set of hierarchical norms operated in Chinese society for the next two thousand years after Dong, although it collapsed when confronted with demands for openness, equality, and freedom of individual human person in the beginning of the twentieth century in China. Does the rejection of entrenched hierarchy in modern societies also imply the irrelevance of Confucian philosophy in our contemporary world? I suggest not, and also that this may prompt us to look elsewhere for Confucian norms, for instance, in the unity of inner sageliness (*neisheng*) and outer kingliness (*waiwang*), that has continuing moral and political significance, and to abandon historically situated norms such as those listed previously.

How do we characterize this political consciousness in Confucianism that starts from a concern and care for the well-being of people and develops into an axiological system of moral virtues? To answer this question, we should reiterate that *ren* is the primary motivating force for the continuing cultivation and transformation of a person in relating to other people. There is no end for such a process of cultivation and transformation since new problems arise, that require constant innovation and vigilance of the self-cultivating person (*junzi*). As Zengzi said in the *Analects*: "It is a heavy task and road is long."[16] It is for this reason that Confucius regards the sage who has perfected the virtue of *ren* as an ideal state of humanity that no living person can be said to reach.

To be mindful of *ren* and to practice it is the first and foremost requirement for government. To govern (*zhi*) is to have power to cause others to follow or obey an order. Hence, a good ruler must know what people want and what is really good for them in order to encourage their trust. This means that, in being a ruler or being in a position to rule, a person must establish himself as a moral person who deserves trust. On the basis of his understanding of the people, Confucius makes this insightful point with regard to political governance. The second requirement for a ruler is that he should have *zhi* or wisdom in conjunction with *ren* so that he is able to make enlightened decisions. A person of *ren* of course also requires a system of *li* (rules of propriety) to make his action sustainable, but this must be made on the basis of the presence of *ren*. In this way, to have *ren* and to conduct oneself correctly in terms of wisdom and moral appropriateness is to conduct oneself as a paradigmatic person whom people can emulate. Thus, Confucius said: "To guide people with virtue and to discipline people with ritual, people will have sense of shame and will come to know how to act right."[17] Thus, if a ruler correctly behaves, people will also act in unison as well. Hence for Confucius, the person who governs has a position like the northern star that is visible to all. There is, however, another essential requirement for good government. The doctrine rectification of names is precisely this requirement; in the Zilu chapter of the *Analects* Confucius said that:

> If names are not rectified, then language will not be smooth, if language is not smooth, things will not be done. If things are not done then rituals and music will not flourish. If rituals and music will not flourish, then punishments will not meet their target. If punishments will not meet their targets, then people do not know what to do.[18]

Correct use of names properly reflects reality but, on the other hand, names are also ways in which we determine what reality is, especially in regard to social and political matters. Here, Confucius requires system of correct names and language that would order social and political relationships as the basis for political administration. His discussion about fathers acting appropriately as fathers should, and sons acting appropriately as sons should, and likewise for rulers and subjects, indicates that there must be established institutions which embody a system of values and which would govern basic human relationships.

Once we have such basic moral and social relationships among people set in order, political order will ensue. Given such a condition, the ruler will simply rule by facing south. This may sound too simplistically idealistic. However, as mentioned previously, in order to reach such a state, the ruler has to set things right beginning with his self-cultivation. Although Confucius did not rule out use of laws of punishment, it was clearly his last resort. What he holds is essentially that we should aim at going above the requirement of law and reaching for the *dao*. Hence he says that the change and reform of the system of Qi could change into the system of Lu and the change and reform of Lu system is then to reach the *dao*. The *dao* here represents the ideal order and harmony of a society that realized the moral relationships of people by way of political maintenance and political exemplification of a moral ruler. The political consciousness of a moral ruler is to hold oneself to the standard of the *dao*.

The idea of rectification (*zheng*) is no doubt the basis for Confucian political consciousness and government. It is the project of transformation of basic morality into political order. It starts with rectification of oneself in cultivating virtues, the essence of which is *ren*. Once the ruler embodies the virtues, he is in a position to institute a system of rules and laws, which would ensure the maintenance of moral relationships among people. The system of rules and laws need not to be laws of punishment, but instead may be understood as constitutive and constitutional as well as regulative and normative. The ruler in his or her wisdom and vision must see to it that such a system of rules and laws is maintained and perhaps modified in times of changing circumstances. This is then the rectification of names based on the rectification of the self of the ruler.[19] We see in the later Confucian document *Daxue* a more detailed description of such a process of transformation of moral order into political order, that is, from self-rectification of a ruler to the rectification of names and ordering of political society.

Is Confucian political philosophy compatible with the modern Western concept of democracy or rule by the people? The answer is ambiguous and depends largely on how we envision the end of political rule. If the end is for social and moral order, insofar as modern democracy will lead to a desirable state of society as conceived by John Dewey, then democracy is compatible with the Confucian political philosophy, including some of its elements of social institutions and infrastructures. On the other hand, if democracy is geared toward political freedom of people to play a significant role in political institutions, then the idea of the benevolent patriarch is indeed a problem. Of course, there is no mention in the Confucian texts of letting people determine how they wish to run their political or public life. The assumption during the Warring States period in China is that people were incapable of making such decisions and therefore needed a wise and benevolent leader to take care of them and to put their lives into order. This is the idea of "Be their ruler and be their teacher."[20] There is also the assumption in Confucianism that people can be directed to do things, but not to know things as noted in the *Analects*. Hence the ruler is given the responsibility to take care of the people for the benefit of the people. On the other hand, the texts also suggest that people can tell a good ruler from a bad ruler and even rise up to remove a bad ruler, as made clear in the *Mencius*. What this ability of people to rise to remove a ruler implies is that the people may select a new ruler. In this sense, part of the Confucian political consciousness of a good ruler is that he must realize that he is a good ruler in the eyes of the people, and, were there an opportunity for the people to exercise political freedom, they would select him. In fact, the Confucian idea of a virtuous ruler is to secure and maintain the trust of the people. The trust of the people is not a matter to be taken lightly as it suggests that the *junzi* must win the trust of the people. That moral cultivation is a prerequisite for political rectitude pushes toward the view that morality lies at the roots of political practice. This transformation would represent a new development of the moral-political philosophy of Confucianism.

Since Confucius advocated self-cultivation for every person, it logically follows that everyone can become a candidate for government. In Confucian literature since the Han, both the idea of selection (*xuan*) and the idea of recommendation (*ju*) have been referred to. The rationale for these methods of selecting someone for a position below oneself, or for accepting a recommendation, was based on the belief in the Mandate of Heaven (*tianming*) as in the *Book of Documents (Shangshu)*. It is of course a narrow view of the process of generating a ruler. However, as Mencius has noted, the *Book of Documents* announce that "Heaven sees through what people see, heaven hears through what people hear."[21] In this statement, the Mandate of Heaven must be founded on the mandate of the people and the Mandate of Heaven is an implicit mandate of people. We must note that for the implicit mandate of people to develop into the democratic consciousness in a modern nation-state, a major step of entrusting people to make a popular election must be made.

Two further observations on Confucian political consciousness can be made. First, in comparison with the Greek city state where people had more active participation in the political affairs of the community, ancient Chinese society was based on an agrarian lifestyle. The people during Confucius' time were primarily engaged with cultivation of land and had to rely on a political order to be constructed on their behalf. Once China becomes more industrialized and people are better educated, the demand for democratic government will undoubtedly be greater. Historically, China as a political entity has been involved in a process of consolidation of political power and integration of an extremely large population. There is also a lack of rational reflection and understanding of the process of succession of political power to the extent that dynastic cycles, by way of intrigue or force, have become a historically entrenched belief among the large majority of Chinese people.

The second observation is this: In the *Annals of Lu (Lu Chunqiu)* in which Confucius praises the moral actions of some dukes and ministers and condemns the immoral behavior and conduct others, he established a tradition of moral critique of political figures in light of their individual actions instead of their institutional practice. This suggests that the political consciousness of Confucianism has subjected a rational consideration of institutions to a moral consideration of personal action. But we do, however, see in Confucius a critical awareness of a need for adaptation for a ritual system and hence a critical awareness of the question of appropriateness and timeliness of a given ritual system or institution in the governance measures implemented by a ruler. This critical awareness may be further developed in conjunction with the notion of accountability of the governing power.

IV. Concluding Remarks

In this article we have dealt with the mainstream schools of Chinese philosophy in the classical period and their contributions to human consciousness in a threefold structure. In the development of these schools, a fundamental consciousness of reality emerges. This is the consciousness of ultimate reality that is the incessant source and foundation for all aspects of Chinese philosophy, including especially the conception of morality and government. But this consciousness of the ultimate that is rooted in a human person can be also described as an original consciousness of reality as a body of truths or a system of truths (*benti*) as experienced by self-conscious individuals. This idea of *benti* has its own inner logic of development as described according to the three levels of human consciousness in Chinese philosophy. In later Chinese intellectual history we see projects that aim to realize emptiness and achieve enlightenment in Chinese Buddhism. We also witness efforts to incorporate Buddhists insights into a Confucian framework as well as those to integrate various strains of thought in new syntheses and formulations of the world and the self. These efforts have continued to the contemporary period and the present day, in the face of larger challenges to understand philosophies on a global and transcultural dimension.

UNIVERSITY OF HAWAII AT MANOA
Honolulu, Hawaii

Endnotes

1. The distinction between the religious and the moral/ethical is such that the former is directed toward stereological beliefs while the latter is directed to rules or virtues of conduct of a person or community in relation to each other.
2. The discovery of Silk Manuscripts with essays on Confucius' understanding of the ancient texts of the *Yijing* was made in 1973 in Mawangdui, Hunan, China. See Deng Qiubai, *Boshu Zhouyi Xiaoshi* (Changsha: Hunan Press, 1987). Edward Shaughnessy made a translation of this text, titled *Book of I Ching* (New York: Ballantine Press, 1997). The discovery of Bamboo Texts on the *Yijing* was made in 1993 in Guodian, Hubei, China. See *Kuodian Chumu Zhujian* (Hubei Jingzhou: Museum Publications, 1973). In 1997 more Bamboo Texts from Hubei were purchased from Hong Kong by the Shanghai Municipal Museum. See *Shanghai Bowuguan Zhushu*, volumes 1 and 2 (Shanghai: Shanghai Museum Publications, 1996–2005).

3. I have pinpointed *"guan"* as represented in the *Yi* text as the foundation and source for developing the system of phenomenal images of nature known as hexagrams. *"Guan"* is a comprehensive viewing and observation of all things in totality in the world from an open and unbiased perspective. This may have to be achieved through a continuous process of observation and reflective integration of experiences. See my essay on *"guan"* in Chung-ying Cheng, *Yixue Benti Lun* [*The* Yi *Ontology*] (Beijing: Beijing University Press, 2006), 77–106.

4. In the "Xici" of the *Yizhuan* we read about how civilization develops and how a sagely ruler becomes enlightening and nourishing like heaven and earth. *Zhouyi Quanjie*, Jin Jingfang and Lu Shaogang, interpretation (Changchun: Jilin University Press, 1996), 445–530; and also see Richard Wilhelm, *The I Ching* (Princeton: Princeton University Press, 1979), 280ff.

5. Of course there were a few creation myths and other mythological legends as recorded in various early texts such as *Chuci, Zhuangzi, Shanhaijing, Huainanzi*. There are also other local myths in minority groups. But there is nothing to compare with the rich repertoire of Greek and Roman mythology or Indic Religion or Nordic Religion as we know them.

6. A few writers are not able to see this distinction. Instead they make a strong contrast between transcendence and immanence which leads to obscuration of the genuine nature of Chinese experience of transcendence. This results in denying a religious dimension of Chinese culture in an effort to impose a Western religious model onto the Chinese experience. We may indeed speak of immanence of human nature as mandate of heaven, but immanence is then conceived as having a dimension of transcendence in the sense I have described as non-exclusive and internal to human experience.

7. See Chung-ying Cheng, "Dimensions of the *Dao* and Onto-ethics in Light of the *DDJ*," *Journal of Chinese Philosophy* 31, no. 2 (2004): 143–82.

8. Refer to Chung-ying Cheng, "On Neville's Understanding of Chinese Philosophy: The Ontology of *Wu*, the Cosmology of *Yi*, and the Normology of *Li*," in *Interpreting Neville*, ed. J. Harley Chapman and Nancy Frankenberry (New York: State University of New York, 1999), 247–70; and Chung-ying Cheng, "On *Dharma* as the *Dao*: A Study of the Transformation of Indian Buddhism into Chinese Philosophy" (paper will be published in the Proceedings of International Conference on Dharma and Abhidharma at Bombay University, Bombay, India, March 14–18, 2005. Forthcoming.

9. Renren Book Series (Taipei: Commercial Press, 1978), vol. 1, 4–14.

10. See the *Analects* of Confucius, Chapter Shuer 7-30. See *Sishu Jizhu*, 78. All translations here and later are by the author.

11. See the *Analects*, Chapter Yanyuan 12-1. See *Sishu Jizhu*, 140.

12. See Chung-ying Cheng, "On *Yi* as a Universal Principle of Specific Application in Confucian Morality," *Philosophy East and West* 22, no. 2 (1972): 269–80.

13. See the *Analects*, Chapter Liren 4-8. See *Sishu Jizhu*, 36.

14. For Mengzi, see *Mengzi, Sishu Jizhu*, commentary by Zhu Xi and explanation by Jiang Boqian (Taipei: Qiming Book Company, 1956), 2a-6, 6a-1, 7a-21. For Xunzi, see *Xunzi Yizhu*, with notes by Gao Changshan (Harbin: Heilongjiang People's Press, 2003), 418. For Daxue, see *Sishu Jizhu*, 1.

15. For Dong's view and philosophy see his work *Chunjiu Fanlu* [*Luxuriant Dews in the Spring and Autumn*]. See Shen Fuwei's *Chunqiu Fanlu Jiaoshi—Shangxiace* [Annotations of Chunqiu Fanlu, 2 volumes] (Baoding: Hebei People's Press, 2005).

16. See *Lunyu*, chaps. 8-7, *Sishu Jizhu*, 86.

17. See the *Analects*, chapter Weizheng 2-3. See *Sishu Jizhu*, 10.

18. See the *Analects*, chapter Zilu 13-3. See *Sishu Jizhu*, 155.

19. See the *Analects*, chapter Yanyuan 12-7 where Confucius says that if a ruler provides leadership in following the rectitude (and hence rectifying oneself with rectitude), no one would dare not to follow rectitude.

20. Mencius has quoted from *Shujing*, "Oath of the Tai," in describing how King Wu regarded the ruler as mandated by heaven as having a sacred mission to lead the people and to enlighten the people. See *Mencius*, Lianghuiwang Chapter, sec. 9. See *Sishu Jizhu*, 29–30.

21. See *Mencius*, Wangzhang Chapter, sec. 5. See *Sishu Jizhu*, 185–87. It is interesting to note that Mencius has combined two requirements for appointing a successor in political power: The ruler has the right to recommend and use a successor, but it is the public opinion and degree of satisfactoriness of the people which is the determinant of whether the appointment is acceptable. This is an implicit affirmation of democracy in a modern sense.

CHINESE GLOSSARY

benti	本體	shen	神
chengyi	誠意	shengsheng	生生
Daodejing	《道德經》	taiji	太極
daqingming	大清明	*Taiji Tushuo*	《太極圖說》
datong	大同	tian	天
Daxue	《大學》	tianming	天命
Dong Zhongshu	董仲舒	tianren heyi	天人合一
fa	法	tianzhi	天志
fajia	法家	tong	同
gu	故	tui	推
guan	觀	waiwang	外王
Han Fei	韓非	wanwu	萬物
hua	化	wu	無
jian	兼	Wudi	武帝
jianai	兼愛	wulun	五倫
jiejuzhidao	絜矩之道	wuwei	無為
ju	舉	"Xiang"	"象"
junzi	君子	xin	心
Laozi	老子	xu	虛
Laozi	《老子》	xuan	选
li	禮	Xunzi	荀子
Liji	《禮記》	yi (creative change)	易
"Liyun"	"禮運"	yi (difference)	異
Lu Chunqiu	《魯春秋》	yi (righteousness)	義
mingde	明德	*Yijing*	《易經》
Mozi	墨子	yin yang	陰陽
neisheng	內聖	*Yizhuan*	《易傳》
qi	氣	yong	勇
ren	仁	yuanqi	元氣
Shangshu	《尚書》	Zengzi	曾子
shangtong	上同	zheng	正

zhi (wisdom)	智	Zhuangzi	莊子
zhi (govern)	治	Zhuxi	朱熹
zhixing heyi	知行合一	Zigong	子貢
Zhongyong	《中庸》	Zilu	子路
Zhou Dunyi	周敦頤	ziran	自然
Zhouyi	《周易》	Zisi	子思

TANG YIJIE

CONSTRUCTING "CHINESE PHILOSOPHY" IN SINO-EUROPEAN CULTURAL EXCHANGE

In December 2002, I published a fourteen-volume series, *Ershi Shiji Xifang Zhexue Dongjian Shi* (*History of the Dissemination of Western Philosophy to China in the 20th Century*).[1] My reason for engaging in this study was to review the history of the importation of Western philosophy into China in order to more fully understand the development of the discipline of "Chinese Philosophy."

There was no such a word as "philosophy," or *zhexue*, in the Chinese language. The term *zhexue* was coined by a Japanese scholar Nishi Amane (1829 97), who borrowed the two Chinese characters *zhe* ("wisdom") and *xue* ("study") to refer to "philosophy" originated in Ancient Greece and Rome. This new term was introduced into China by a Chinese scholar, Huang Zunxian (1848–1905), and was accepted by Chinese scholars. Although this term *zhexue* was accepted by Chinese scholars late in the nineteenth century, the problem remained, regarding whether China had "philosophy" or the sort that was comparable to Western philosophy. Indeed, this issue is still being debated by contemporary scholars in the field.

Western philosophy was imported into China at the end of the nineteenth century. Its foremost and most influential introducer, Yan Fu (1853–1921), had translated numerous Western philosophical texts into Chinese, especially those pertaining to evolutionary theory. In quick succession, the texts of Kant, Descartes, Schopenhauer, and Nietzsche were introduced into China. These movements provided a perspective on the issue of whether there is philosophy in China. Some Chinese scholars discovered that although "philosophy" was not an independent discipline, there were ample philosophical themes and questions in the classical Chinese canons, such as *Shang Shu* (*Book of History*), *Yi Jing* (*Book of Changes*), *Lun Yu* (Confucian *Analects*), *Lao Zi*, and *Zhuang Zi*, that were comparable to those in Western philosophy. There were also significant differ-

TANG YIJIE, Professor, Peking University and President of the Academy of Chinese Culture. Specialties: history of Chinese philosophy, classical Confucian texts, Chinese Buddhist philosophy. E-mail: tyjydy@pku.edu.cn

ences between the inquiries in these canons and those in Western philosophy, and study of these differences were invaluable to scholarship.

We must acknowledge that, before the importation of Western philosophy, there was no scholarly study of Chinese philosophy in its own right, as a field distinct from "canon studies" (*jing xue*) and "traditions of the masters" (*zi xue*). From the first half of the twentieth century, there was a surge into China of the fields of Western philosophy including Marxism, Pragmatism, Realism, Analytic Philosophy, Ancient Greek Philosophy, and nineteenth-century German Philosophy. This had a powerful impact on scholarship in China. As a result of their engagement with Western philosophy and its frameworks, Chinese scholars attempted to compile voluminous collections of classical canons and commentaries associated with Kongzi (Confucius), Laozi, Zhuangzi, and so forth, in order to establish a discipline of "Chinese philosophy." In the early stages, such study focused only on the thoughts of particular individuals or isolated topics. By the twentieth century, however, the field of Chinese philosophy had been founded primarily through the route of studies in Chinese intellectual history. During this period, several volumes of "History of Chinese Philosophy," including Hu Shih's (Hu Shi) *Zhongguo Zhexue Shi Dagang* (*Outline of the History of Chinese Philosophy*[2]) and Feng Youlan's (Fung Yu-lan) *Zhongguo Zhexue Shi* (*History of Chinese Philosophy*[3]), were authored by scholars who sought to demonstrate that Chinese philosophy had pre-Qin (before 221 BCE) origins. In other words, these Chinese thinkers were consciously separating philosophical study from studies in classics and studies under masters, and establishing Chinese philosophy as an independent disciplinary field. Nevertheless, all these accounts of Chinese intellectual history were greatly influenced and defined by the frameworks supplied by Western philosophy.

From the 1930s, Chinese philosophers were absorbing and adapting Western philosophy in their accounts of Chinese philosophy. This led to the articulation of several modern versions of Chinese philosophy. The prominent thinkers of this period include Xiong Shili, Zhang Dongsun, Feng Youlan, and Jin Yuelin. Unfortunately, after 1949, such attempts to construct strains of modern Chinese philosophy were abruptly halted, as were studies that sought to engage dialogue between Chinese and Western philosophies.

It was not until the 1980s, when China embraced reforms toward a more open society, that the study of Chinese philosophy was again permitted. The doctrines of existentialism, Western Marxism, phenomenology, structuralism, hermeneutics, postmodernism, semiotics, to name a few, were introduced in China. This not only broadened the horizons of Chinese philosophers, but also provided many different perspectives for richer, in-depth scholarship in Chinese philosophy.

From this brief retrospective on the history of the importation of Western philosophy into China, I would like to make the following proposals in order to generate further discussion.

I. Western Philosophy and Chinese Philosophy as an Independent Discipline

There was neither an original Chinese term *zhexue* nor did Chinese philosophy as an independent discipline originate in China. It was only in engagement with and response to Western philosophy that elements of philosophical ideas and philosophical questions were identified in the Chinese classics. Hence, the "Chinese philosophy" that had been developed through this period was primarily constructed according to paradigms and frameworks provided by Western philosophy. Take Feng Youlan's *History of Chinese Philosophy* for example. Its structure, terminology, and perspectives were mainly borrowed from their equivalents in Western philosophy. These include concepts such as idealism and materialism, ontology and cosmology, monism and dualism (or pluralism), empirical and transcendental, phenomenon and essence, universals and particulars, thought and existence, and the like. These conceptual frameworks were employed to explain certain notions in Chinese thought including *dao*, *tian*, and *xin*. Existing ideas, issues, terminologies, concepts, and logic were shaped by Western philosophy. Fortuitously, the result was greater clarity in the specification of issues and outline of concepts, as well as greater precision in logic. I suggest that this was a necessary step in the creation of a viable "Chinese philosophy."

Modern Chinese philosophy of the 1930s and 1940s is comprised by scholarly work that characteristically *continues* rather than *follows* the traditional discourse of Chinese philosophy. That is to say, in the process of studying and adapting Western philosophy, Chinese philosophers transformed Chinese philosophy from the traditional to the modern. This continued development in Chinese philosophy had to meet the criteria of Western philosophy; attempt to "converge the Chinese and the West" was primarily involved supplementing the shortcomings of Chinese scholarship with those of Western scholarship. Let me demonstrate this with two representative examples. The first is Xiong Shili's doctrine of the Neo-Weishi Lun (Yogācāra Buddhism),[4] and the second Feng Youlan's Neo-Confucianism (*xin lixue*).[5]

Xiong Shili's Neo-Weishi Lun is only partially complete. The completed section, the "Doctrine of the Jing" (*jing lun*), is a treatise that covers topics in the field of ontology (*benti lun*) in Western philosophy, albeit with some Chinese characteristics. The other section which he had originally planned to write was the "Doctrine of the Liang" (*liang lun*). Had it been written, this section would have covered a topic area roughly equivalent to epistemology (*renshi lun*) in Western philosophy. His other works allow us a glimpse as well into his view of Chinese philosophy as it stands in relation to Western philosophy. Xiong believes that traditional Chinese philosophy tended to place more emphasis on experiential wisdom (*tiren*) than rational judgment or analysis (*sibian*). For Xiong, this is where discussions on epistemology in Western philosophy can benefit Chinese philosophy: He envisaged an epistemological approach that synthesized experiential wisdom with rational analysis.

In his approach to Neo-Confucianism, Feng Youlan asserts that his vision was not to follow, but to continue, the Neo-Confucianism of the Song (960–1280) and the Ming (1368–1644) Dynasties. Feng's approach resulted in an introduction into Chinese philosophy the "universals" (*gong xiang*) and "particulars" (*shu xiang*) of Platonic philosophy, as well as ideas in Neo-Realism (*xin shizai lun*). Using this schema, the world is divided into "truth" (*zhenji*)—or principle (*li*) or great ultimate (*taiji*)—and "reality" (*shiji*). Accordingly, things in reality become what they are according to their essence or principle. In adapting the bipolar concepts of truth and reality, Feng was able to continue the Neo-Confucian doctrine of the "many sharing the one" (*li yi fen shu*). Another Neo-Confucian work of Feng Youlan, entitled *A New Understanding of Words* (*Xin Zhi Yan*),[6] discusses philosophical methodology and its relation to epistemological questions. According to Feng, Western philosophy excels in analysis while traditional Chinese philosophy excels in intuition. His treatment of Neo-Confucianism combines, and reaps the benefits of, both these approaches.

Both Xiong Shili and Feng Youlan drew from traditional Chinese thought to articulate Chinese philosophy. However, they continued the tradition by taking on Western philosophy as the fundamental framework. Unfortunately, such exciting developments in Chinese philosophy were forestalled by external circumstances.

From the discussion above, it is clear that whether we understand Chinese philosophy in terms of its early forays into Chinese intellectual history or its continuing development in the early modern period in Chinese history, we must recognize that it was very much shaped by Western philosophy.

II. Paradigms and Frameworks of Western Philosophy and Potential Problems in Chinese Philosophy

As humans, we inevitably share a number of common characteristics that cut across different civilizations and cultures. Nevertheless, each civilization or culture is unique in geographical, historical, and even accidental aspects. Naturally, we expect that Western philosophy will have distinctive characteristics due to its evolution within a particular sociocultural environment. Likewise, Chinese philosophy will necessarily be influenced by social and cultural factors and hence will possess certain particularities. Thus, injudicious and unrestrained construction of Chinese philosophy according to the terms of reference in Western philosophy will unavoidably be problematic. I believe there are at least two fundamental problems.

The first problem concerns the obliteration of characteristics of Chinese philosophy that may be of unique significance to philosophical inquiry. I will discuss two key features of Chinese philosophy that will help to demonstrate this point. Western philosophy from the time of the ancient Greeks and especially from Descartes on, has regarded more highly the systematic construction of philosophic knowledge. By contrast, thinkers in the Chinese tradition have put more emphasis on the pursuit of certain paths or goals in order to realize one's virtue or efficacy (*jingshen jingjie*). A passage in the Confucian *Analects* portrays Confucius' emphasis on the "inner," personal pleasure associated with learning: "The Master said, 'They who know the truth are not equal to those who love it, and they who love it are not equal to those who delight in it'" (*Analects* 6:18).[7] The ultimate pursuit of life is not merely to attain knowledge or acquire skills; Yan Hui, Confucius' much loved disciple, harmonized his love of learning and personal conduct (*Analects* 6:3). In Yan Hui, the body and mind, the exterior and the interior, were in harmony.

The Daoist philosopher Zhuangzi pursued *jingshen jingjie* of spontaneous wandering in his first chapter, "Xiaoyao you,"[8] that was not cramped by conventional aspirations and values. Similarly, a well-known Chan Buddhist poem articulates the *jingshen jingjie* of being comfortable in different environments:

> The spring flowers, the autumn moon;
> Summer breezes, winter snow.
> If useless things do not clutter your mind,
> You have the best days of your life.[9]

The spirit of such a philosophy characterized by reflective personal engagement with its insights is distinct from those predominant in Western philosophy, but its value for humanity cannot be underestimated.

Another distinctive and fundamental characteristic of traditional Chinese thought is its balance of holistic and individual perspectives. The key notions in traditional Chinese philosophy include "the unity of heaven and humanity" (*tian ren he yi*), "the myriad of things are one" (*wanwu yiben*) and "the unity of body and mind, the exterior and the interior" (*shenxin neiwai heyi*). These fundamental paradigms stand in contrast to the subject-orientated approaches and the subject–object dichotomy that are dominant in (Western) Anglo-analytic philosophy. If this subject-orientation and its attendant dualistic frameworks are used as reference points from which to understand Chinese philosophy, the distinctive characteristics of the latter will not be sufficiently articulated. On the other hand, it is important to note that the themes in Chinese philosophy outlined above are more closely aligned in spirit and approach with those in continental European philosophy, such as, for instance, in Phenomenology, which emphasizes the intersubjective nature (*hu zhu ti xing*) of an individual's engagement with the world. To bring to the foreground these features in traditional Chinese thinking will benefit both Chinese and Western philosophies.

The second source of potential problems is related to the translation of Chinese terms and phrases into English. There are many notions in traditional Chinese thought such as *tian, dao, xin, xing, you, wu,* and *qi,* with distinctive meanings within specific philosophical frameworks that are difficult to express in correspondence with Western philosophy. For example, *tian* (often "thinly" translated "Heaven") has at least three meanings:

(a) supreme and ultimate heaven, some times expressed in terms of a personal god;
(b) naturalistic heaven that incorporates a sense of the natural environment; and
(c) heaven associated with a transcendent order; this is the ground of normative principles (*yili*) that may also have implications for ethical conduct.

Another example is *qi,* which may be interpreted in at least three ways:

(a) material existence;
(b) vitality and consciousness, as for instance in Mencius' and energetic and dynamic *qi* (*huo qi zhi qi*) or the *Guanzi*'s essential *qi* (*jing qi*); or
(c) the ultimate, as for instance in the "one *qi* evolved into three" (*yiqi hua sanqing*) theme in Daoist thought.

It is not easy to find parallels to all these meanings of *qi* in Western philosophy. Strictly speaking, some of them cannot be translated, and

I suggest in these cases to use transliterations. Here, I refer to an example of successful use of transliteration in order to preserve the original insights of a doctrine. When Buddhist thought was introduced into China, several important notions including "prajna" (*banruo*) and "nirvana" (*niepan*) were only transliterated. In time, these transliterations were adopted into the Chinese language, and their original Indian Buddhist meanings were retained. It is important to note that the Dharma exponent, Xuan Zang (600–664), deliberately articulated five principles of "no translation" (*wu bufan*) in relation to the concepts in the Buddhist canons.[10] We may follow this example to sustain the potency and uniqueness of certain distinctive notions in Chinese philosophy, rather than assimilate them according to Western terminologies. However, some indiscriminate superimpositions of categories and paradigms in Western philosophy have already reduced the amplitude and distinctiveness of several concepts in Chinese thought. There is a need to handle these concepts carefully, including attending to translation and transliteration issues so as not to erroneously circumscribe them. Careful consideration of these issues will enhance the contribution of Chinese philosophy to contemporary philosophical debates.

III. Future Developments in Chinese Philosophy

In my view, scholars of Chinese philosophy should continue serious and systematic study of Western philosophy, paying special attention to its new trends. In particular, these new developments reflect concerns about globalization and its implications for human understanding, advances in science and technology and their impact on the environment, moral development, and conceptions of human well-being, to name a few. Here, I make a suggestion for future research.

I draw upon the history of the adaptation and synthesis of Buddhism into Chinese culture to illustrate how we might approach the engagement of Chinese and Western philosophies. During the Sui and Tang Dynasties (from the sixth to the eighth centuries), several sinicized Buddhist schools emerged in China. These schools developed the doctrines of Indian Buddhism by integrating within it Confucian and Daoist ideas.

In engaging Chinese and Western philosophies, one important methodological approach is to employ relevant themes and concepts in Chinese thought to explicate and embellish ideas in Western philosophy. This kind of study not only broadens the scope of Western philosophy, but also makes new contributions to the discipline of philosophy. We are now aware that this is an emergent approach as, for instance, in the theses of scholars who discuss Chinese hermeneutics, Chinese phenomenology, Chinese semiotics, and the like. In this light, the phrase "Chinese philosophy" should apply not only to "the philosophy of the Chinese," but also to philosophy that influences contemporary debates in a distinctive way.

This method is compatible with the kind of constructive strategy used by a number of Chinese scholars in the 1930s and 1940s, which I had referred to earlier. Scholars including Xiong Shili and Feng Youlan constructed the early Chinese philosophical traditions in resonance with Western philosophical themes and concepts to create a modern Chinese philosophy. Indeed, scholars now may even extend and continue the work of Xiong Shili and Feng Youlan, just as they continue the traditions of Confucius, Mencius, Zhu Xi, and Wang Yangming in their engagement with Western philosophy. In brief, scholars in the field of Chinese philosophy should both take up the standpoint of its proper tradition and effectively absorb and adapt new ideas in contemporary Western philosophy. In contemporary Chinese–Western cultural exchange we should, in our dialogues, place these philosophies on equal footing. This will allow philosophical discussions to achieve significant developments in the twenty-first century. Active engagement in these discussions will enhance the development of philosophy, Chinese and Western, in an increasingly globalized world.

PEKING UNIVERSITY
Beijing, China

ENDNOTES

1. Tang Yijie, ed., *History of the Dissemination of Western Philosophy to China in the 20th Century* [*Ershi Shiji Xifang Zhexue Dongjian Shi*], 14 vols. (Beijing: Shoudu shifan daxue chubanshe, 2002).
2. Hu Shih, *Outline of the History of Chinese Philosophy* (Beijing: Dong Fang Press, 1996), originally entitled *History of Pre-Qin Sophism* [*Xian Qin Mingxue Shi*], written between 1915 and 1917 and first published in 1922.
3. Feng Youlan, *History of Chinese Philosophy*, vol. 1 (first published in 1931) and vol. 2 (first published in 1934) (Beijing: Zhong Hua Shuju, 1962).
4. Tang Yijie and Xiao Jiefu, eds., *Xiong Shili Lunzhu Ji Zhiyi: Xin Weishi Lun* [*Collected Works of Xiong Shili [1]: New Doctrine of Consciousness Only*] (Beijing: Zhonghua Shuju, 1985).
5. Feng Youlan, *Xin Li-xue* [*New Rational Philosophy*] (Changsha: Commercial Press, 1939).
6. Feng Youlan, *Xin zhi yan* [*A New Understanding of Words*] (Shanghai: Commercial Press, 1946).
7. James Legge, trans., *The Four Books* (Taiwan: Culture Book Company, 1981), 195. The following quotations from this book will show chapter and page number(s) in parenthesis.

8. Angus C. Graham, trans., *Chuang-Tzu: The Inner Chapters* (Indianapolis: Hackett, 2001), 43–47. Graham translates "Xiaoyao you" as "Going Rambling with a Destination."

9. Wumen Huikai (Mumon Ekai), *The Gateless Gate* (Wumen guan in Chinese; Mumonkan in Japanese). English translation by Katsuki Sekida, *Two Zen Classics: The Gateless Gate and the Blue Cliff Records* (Boston: Shambhala Press, 2005, previously published in 1995 by Weatherhill Press). Translation available online at http://www.sacred-texts.com/bud/zen/mumonkan.htm (accessed on February 23, 2007).

10. According to the Song Dynasty scholar Zhou Dunyi, Xuan Zang's *wu bufan* recommends that Sanskrit terms should only be transliterated, rather than translated, in the following five situations: the terms are arcane, such as in incantations; they have multiple meanings; there are no equivalent terms in Chinese; traditionally these terms have been transliterated and not translated; and if translation might obscure a profound concept. (Zhou Dunyi, *Fanyi Minyi Xu* [*Preface to the Explanation of Buddhist Terms*] [Beijing: Shangwu Yinshuguan, 1984], 54.1055).

Chinese Glossary

banruo	般若	*Lun Yu*	《论语》
benti lun	本体论	niepan	涅槃
dao	道	qi	气
Ershi Shiji Xifang Zhexue Dongjian Shi	《二十世纪西方哲学东渐史》	renshi lun	认识论
		Shang Shu	《尚书》
Fanyi Minyi Xu	《翻譯名義序》	shenxin neiwai heyi	身心内外合一
Feng Youlan	冯友兰	shiji	实际
gong xiang	共相	shu xiang	殊相
Guanzi	《管子》	sibian	思辨
Huang Zunxian	黄遵宪	taiji	太极
huo qi zhi qi	活气之气	tian	天
Hu Shi	胡适	tiren	休认
hu zhu ti xing	互主体性	wanwu yiben	万物一本
jing lun	境论	weishi	唯识
jing qi	精气	wu	无
jingshen jingjie	精神境界	wu bufan	五不翻
jing xue	经学	Wumen Huikai	無門慧開
Jin Yuelin	金岳霖	*Xian Qin Mingxue Shi*	《先秦名学史》
Lao Zi	《老子》	"Xiaoyao you"	"逍遥游"
li	理	xin	心
liang lun	量论	xing	性
li yi fen shu	理一分殊	xin lixue	新理学

xin shizai lun	新实在论	zhenji	真际
Xin Zhi Yan	《新知言》	zhexue	哲学
Xiong Shili	熊十力	*Zhuang Zi*	《庄子》
Xuan Zhuang	玄奘	*Zhongguo Zhexue Shi*	
Yan Fu	严复	《中国哲学史》	
Yi Jing	《易经》	*Zhongguo Zhexue Shi Dagang*	
yili	义理	《中国哲学史大纲》	
yiqi hua sanqing	一气化三清	Zhou Dunyi	周敦義
you	有	zi xue	子学
Zhang Dongsun	张东荪		

NATHAN SIVIN

DRAWING INSIGHTS FROM CHINESE MEDICINE

Research on science and medicine has often pointed my way toward understanding how certain key themes in Chinese philosophy evolved.[1] I therefore wish to suggest why attention to recent insights in the history of Chinese medicine can lead to new perceptions about thought in general. The physical sciences are as useful as medicine for this purpose, but that is another topic.

I. Han Thought

In the past fifteen years, a new way of looking at the late Warring States and Han eras has swept away a host of sinological platitudes. I will review a couple of these changes that involve medicine and philosophy. One is the uncomfortable issue of schools; the second, a natural corollary of that, is the fate of that slippery item "Huang-Lao Daoism" on the philosophical agenda.

II. "Schools"

Students of Chinese thought for generations have used the term "school" to convince each other that their disembodied analyses of texts fit somewhere, somehow, in society. These days the word "school," if it appears at all, tends to sit inside quotation marks, to signal an uneasy choice of words. But the picture is now clear enough that the notion of "school" can be discarded once and for all.

"School" in modern sinological usage is almost always equivalent to the twentieth-century Chinese term *xuepai*. There is no corresponding word in ancient writing. Closest to a counterpart is *jia*. But *jia* originally meant not a collegial body but a family: The place they live and those who live there. Over the last five years, half a dozen scholars have shown that Sima Tan (d. 110 BC) borrowed this familial notion of *jia* to stand not for people, but for trends of thought. While constructing a highly partisan argument for his political viewpoint, he

NATHAN SIVIN, Professor Emeritus of Chinese Culture and of the History of Science, University of Pennsylvania. Specialities: history of Chinese thought, Chinese religion, science and medicine. E-mail: nsivin@sas.upenn.edu

applied this word for the first time to six categories of thought, including three brand new ones, those of names (*mingjia*), laws (*fajia*), and yinyang (*yingyangjia*). This argument was not meant to be an objective historical analysis. Misreading it as one—a careless mistake common among twentieth-century historians of thought—has generated many misconceptions about the social organization of ancient philosophy.

Before Sima's essay, surveys of philosophy had been about masters and how they embodied their teachings and passed them down. The well-known attacks on rivals by Xunzi and others were polemics against people, not against abstract concepts.[2] Sima's use of *jia* was so original and counterintuitive that no writer on philosophy in the Han followed it; the issue remained people and their embodiment of teachings.[3] In philosophy, *jia* came to mean a lineage (like a family line) that claimed descent from a single master. Usually the presumed founder of each lineage was an ancient sage, his teachings transmitted in a written text that one's own teacher explained, with a solemn ritual of initiation.[4] Liu Xiang (79–8 BC) and his son Liu Xin (46 BC–AD 23) later introduced a quite different focus, on books rather than people. When they catalogued the imperial library that they largely created, they made *jia* a counter for one book title—not one conception or one author—and also for subdivisions of one of its bibliographic categories. As Sarah Queen put it, "approaching their inventories as accurate descriptions of the prominent traditions of the Han era is to misread them and miss their polemical nuances."[5]

By the end of the Han period, roughly AD 200, the vitality of philosophic lineages was largely gone.[6] If *jia* means a long-lasting textual tradition embodied in identifiable masters and disciples, none but Confucian lineages outlasted the Han period. What gave them their standing was not the outcome of debates, but an imperial edict in 136 BC that ended the appointment of officials to teach other ancient books. Among those no longer taught, for instance, was Confucius' *Analects*. This edict was the outcome of intense political infighting, not of sagely reflection.[7]

To sum up this point, for Chinese philosophy from the Han period on, *jia* in most cases has meant a tradition of textual transmission and a belief in common descent. It does not imply a school in any social or architectural sense.

III. HUANG-LAO

The Huang-Lao bandwagon came rolling out of the excavations at Mawangdui in the years following 1973. Tang Lan in 1974 claimed that four Mawangdui manuscripts were actually the lost *Four Classics of the Yellow Emperor* (*Huangdi Si Jing*).[8] A number of his colleagues agreed. A few American sinologists uncritically gave the doctrine of the "four classics" a clear-cut status in philosophical history as "Huang-Lao Daoism"—as usual, without defining "Daoism." Not all of them noticed the point of Tang's exercise: In the circumstances of the Great Proletarian Cultural Revolution, to present a politically correct view of, as he put it, the "struggle between the Confucians and the Legalists in early Han."[9]

The bandwagon sped along until, from the middle 1990s on, one specialist after another has acknowledged that these texts cannot be the *Four Classics* after all.[10] In fact, we cannot reliably identify any excavated text with records of early Yellow Emperor writings. Some time in the past five years, the bandwagon finally creaked to a halt in the middle of nowhere.

The result was a setback with respect to understanding the Huangdi tradition. But there was no reason to be pessimistic. The main reason for our ignorance of Huangdi was what I think of as the Awesome Taboo. By that I mean the custom among European and American sinologists of never, ever, reading any old scientific or medical text, or even opening one, under threat of penalties so dreadful that no one has ever said what they are. The reign of this dreadful prohibition seems to have begun gradually in the twentieth century. Western students of China up to that time tended to be more broadly competent, and to have been healthily curious about their subjects' views of nature and the human body. The Awesome Taboo never affected Chinese and Japanese scholars. In the West it has finally begun to die out as students no longer fear and disdain science. With that in mind, we can move on to medicine.

IV. MEDICINE AND THE HAN PHILOSOPHICAL SYNTHESES

Young sinologists are now reading books of central importance in early thought that the Awesome Taboo prevented their elders from opening. Until recently, histories of philosophy in European languages ignored or barely mentioned the *Spring and Autumn Annals of Master Lu* (*Lu Shi Chunqiu*, 239/235 BC) and the *Supreme Mystery* (*Tai Xuan Jing*, c. 4 BC).[11]

From the Han Dynasty on, many scholars believed that the *Changes* (*Yi Jing*) is an infallible guide to change in the cosmos because its structure is the structure of cosmic process.[12] Today we are aware of that those scholars read the structure into it. But readers now find in the *Supreme Mystery* what later scholars read into the

Changes. Yang Xiong shaped his book into a poetic, systematic scheme of cyclic change in the cosmos.

Among the astonishing riches of the *Springs and Autumns of Master Lu*, readers find a sophisticated theoretical schema of the human body, its functions, and its dysfunctions—something not found in the Mawangdui manuscripts, and not in any medical book for another 150 years or so. The book's early integration of medicine with philosophy alerts open-minded readers to three long and important Yellow Emperor books that have been there all along.

Despite their conceptual depth, no author on Chinese philosophy in previous generations has analyzed three early, indubitable Yellow Emperor classics devoted to medicine. These three have been copied, printed, and reprinted for nearly two thousand years, can be found in every Chinese library, and for the past millennium have been familiar to every learned physician and a great many laymen: the *Yellow Emperor's Inner Canon* (*Huangdi Nei Jing*, probably first century BC); the *Canon of 81 Problems [in the Inner Canon] of the Yellow Emperor* (*Huangdi Bashiyi Nan Jing*, probably second century AD); and the *"A-B" Canon of the Yellow Emperor* (*Huangdi Jiayi Jing*, 256/282).[13] The first of these is a jumble of short texts; the second and third are early attempts to impose order and consistency on them.[14]

Now what do these books tell us about the mysterious Huang-Lao—that is, the Yellow Emperor and Laozi? Actually, they have nothing at all to say about Laozi, just as the *Laozi* has nothing to say about Huangdi. But these medical texts cast much light on the Yellow Emperor.

The *Inner Canon* is a collection of dialogues between the Yellow Emperor and his various ministers. In most of these short texts, his courtiers are also his teachers. When the emperor turns to what we think of today as the internal organs, he asks to hear "about the relative authority of the functions associated with the viscera, about which is higher in rank and which lower."[15] He assumes, in other words, that the body, like the state, is a bureaucracy. His instructor systematically spells out the details, with the heart as ruler, and the rest of the somatic functions dependent on how the heart nourishes its vital forces.

The chapter closes with a moral for the monarch. What the heart does for the body, it says, is exactly what the ruler contributes to government. By ceaseless self-cultivation he makes his oversight sagely, and leaves running the state to his ministers. As early sources tell us, that is a fundamental principle of the Yellow Emperor's teachings.[16] In other such discussions, in the *Inner Canon* and other books, not only is the body a state, but the state is a body. It is not that one furnishes metaphors for the other; as parts of a whole they spontaneously correspond. The physician, like the Yellow Emperor, keeps body processes in harmony with those of heaven and earth. The sage ruler does the same thing for the processes of governance.

Again, just as the state was a small cosmos, the sky was a large state. The area surrounding the pole star was the imperial palace, and astronomers recognized four other portions of the sky as local courts. The *Book of Celestial Offices* (*Tian Guan Shu*), a treatise in *Records of the Grand Astrologer*, lists the constellations as civil service departments staffed by stars.[17]

In other words, the *Inner Canon* and the other Yellow Emperor classics tell us about a unity that encompassed the state, the cosmos, and the human body. Cosmology, ritual, morality, rulership, and divination were ways to understand and act on that unity. In normal circumstances, the vital rhythms of all three domains were in perfect harmony. Medicine deals with disturbances in that order within the body (*bing, ji*); statecraft deals with disorder in society (*luan*). Sagely doctors and sagely rulers repair both with the same action, *zhi*, "ordering."

We can now see that the unity I am discussing supported social authority and political power. That is hardly surprising. From Lu Buwei (c. 291–235 BC) on, the same intellectuals set the standards in all three domains: cosmology, political theory, and medical doctrine. They made the empire possible, but at the same time they tried to limit the power of the ruler by urging him to be a ritualist and meditator rather than an activist.

In other words, the medical canon, like the *Supreme Mystery*, lets us see a mature form of a philosophy—natural, somatic, political, social—that had been slowly evolving for centuries. *It provides a more comprehensive account of that philosophy than any other Han book.* Its synthesis and that of the *Supreme Mystery* provided a stable starting point for later thought to build on.

Several enterprising scholars, including Wang Aihe, Michael Nylan, Sarah Queen, Mark Csikszentmihalyi, and Kidder Smith, are studying the evolution I have mentioned.[18] They are beginning to make sense of the political rivalries and confrontations of ideals that Han philosophic and medical writings reflect. To accomplish that requires reading ancient Chinese texts as assertions of individuals with interests, ideals, ambitions, frustrations, and prejudices rather than as objective, authoritative pronouncements. The most capable sinologists have been doing that for a long time. The innovation lies in a style of interpretation deeply informed by the insights of anthropology, sociology, religious studies, and modern philosophy.

V. The Meaning of the Han Syntheses

Now what insights do these old technical treatises and new inquiries prompt? Some years ago I published an essay entitled "On the Word 'Taoism' as a Source of Perplexity."[19] It offered a simple observation and a modest proposal. It observed that scholars who wrote about Daoism tended to use the word in as many as twenty senses, sometimes shifting among three or four different meanings in the same paragraph. This was true of various other "isms" as well, above all of Confucianism.

In sinology, there is no possibility of agreeing on a single definition of anything. I simply suggested that when people write about Daoism or Confucianism, in each case they just say explicitly what they mean by the word. Having read in a recent issue of the *Journal of Chinese Philosophy* an article that gave not just one definition of Confucianism but four,[20] I have some reason to hope that my proposal will eventually prove to be useful.

I might add that, as a personal experiment, for some years I tried doing entirely without "isms" when I wrote about thought. Whenever I was tempted to mention Daoism or something similar, instead I just asked myself which persons I was thinking about, and wrote about them instead. The result, I think, has been a clear gain in clarity and cogency. That experiment encouraged me to see the Yellow Emperor doctrines of the Han in a larger setting than any "ism" offers. No doubt the important theme of the emperor as a quietist rather than an activist is abstractly related to the notion of *wuwei*, or "non-purposive action," in the *Laozi*. But when Ban Gu in the *History of the Former Han Dynasty* (*Qian Hanshu*) praised the emperor Wen for not getting in the way of his large and active bureaucracy, that was hardly what the authors of the *Laozi* were writing about.[21]

In the same way, what I find most striking about what some historians call Han Confucianism is how many of Confucius' central teachings those who claimed to be strict Confucians rejected. First, there was his humanism—the conviction that the problems of the good life are fundamentally moral, to be overcome only in the domain of the person and his relations to others. To his quest non-human nature and the cosmos were irrelevant. Han thinkers from Lu Buwei on rejected this humanism. They averred that the sagely life has to be in step with the rhythms that govern heaven, earth, and the state. The emperor, responsible for that linkage, was a sage by virtue of his office. They made cosmology a key to social order, individual cultivation, and effective action. How about the successful argument of Dong Zhongshu and others in 136 BC that the government should regulate which books were to be taught, in line with the needs of state security? That justification hardly would have occurred to Confucius.

This list of rejections could be much longer, but I think the point is clear. There was no single Han synthesis, but there was a succession of competing ones. They shared several characteristics: They freely revised and combined almost every philosophic viewpoint circulating in their time. Which came from Laozi and which from Confucius ceased to matter. They fitted all of them into a larger scheme based on a unity of the cosmos, the state, and the healthy individual body. Their schemata solidly underpinned the legitimacy of the imperial state. They incorporated an analytical language based on yinyang, *wuxing* (the five phases), and *qi*. In the *Inner Canon* and the *Supreme Mystery*, these concepts attained the relationship they kept for two thousand years afterward. *Qi* had become the basic stuff of the cosmos, and the vitality that maintained processes and made change happen. Yinyang and the five phases provided equivalent ways of dividing *qi*, twofold and fivefold, in order to understand the aspects of a total process or configuration.[22]

These syntheses ended most of the lineages of transmission that had kept other classics alive. In that sense, the *Analects*, the *Laozi*, the *Zhuangzi*, the *Mozi*, and any number of others practically ceased to exist as distinct intellectual forces until, in later centuries, other thinkers revived them for new philosophic, religious, or political enterprises—for instance, when ritualists of an early Daoist community reinvented Laozi as a superhuman savior.[23] I am necessarily oversimplifying a complicated story. Still, it does not make sense to treat the Han teachings as timeless essences in some immaterial space. They were intended to create a lasting imperium, and they succeeded.

The Huang-Lao Daoism debacle of the last generation grew directly out of some sinologists' longing to find a missing link, any vague kind of link, between the old Daoism of *wuwei* and paradox, and the new post-Han Daoist movements with their hereditary priesthoods, their innumerable gods, and their search for imperial patronage. This longing was based on a faith that, since specialists call both Daoisms, they must be linked. The tail, in other words, was wagging the dog. The debacle turned out to be a mere distraction from the rich Huangdi medical texts waiting to be studied as key documents of Han philosophy, neither Confucian nor Daoist in any meaningful sense.

I have suggested one kind of insight that acquaintance with early medicine can yield. Looking from this unfamiliar point of view at what philosophy became in the Han may make that momentous transition a little clearer.

VI. Medicine and Philosophy after the Han

The study of medicine can be useful in many other ways. We could look at recent work on how books took the forms we know, beginning in the late Warring States period. That research is clearing up a great deal of confusion about when as well as how the books we explore today came into being. This line of investigation took its first large step, it happens, with a remarkable study of the *Inner Canon of the Yellow Emperor* in the dissertation of David Keegan in 1988. Maruyama Masao and Ma Jixing also made important independent contributions. This work too has notably accelerated in the past decade.[24]

The opportunities to apply insights from medicine to post-Han philosophy are just as rich. A recent volume edited by Hsiung Pingchen directly compares published medical case records (*yian*) with books on transmission in Confucian lineages (*xuean*), throwing light on the origins of the latter.[25] Or we might look at Wu Yiyi's reconstruction of how learning passed down a single medical lineage for three hundred years, from the twelfth to the fifteenth century. Wu's analysis reveals how the mode of transmission changed over this long period, and in particular the great and permanent influence of printing and the book trade. People who study philosophical teachings can easily use his methodology.

We could also explore philosophy *in* medicine. Some historians of medicine, when they discuss physicians, use the adjective "Confucian" with great abandon. The term "*ru* physician" (*ruyi*) was coined by palace officials in 1103 as part of a new educational policy that would tempt sons of elite families to study medicine.[26] As we would expect, not many people so labeled were Confucians in the strict sense—trained and initiated in a line of textual transmission. There were a few. The most notable of these was Zhu Zhenheng (1282–1358), one of the four celebrated physicians who moved medicine in new directions in the Song and Yuan periods.[27] No one has yet looked into what the practice of the real Confucian healers had in common, or how they differed from the rank and file of elite physicians. There is also a quickly growing literature that applies the *Book of Changes* to medical doctrine and studies the many early books that did the same thing.[28] That topic needs research from a sophisticated philosophical point of view. There is, in a word, no shortage of opportunities for ground-breaking research.

I sometimes hear from sinologist colleagues who would like to look into early medical literature, but who expect it to be terribly hard to read. To the contrary, its technical content tends to be simple in form and syntax. When I first began studying classical medicine, I did find its terminology difficult, since the dictionaries ignored the medical classics, and there were no reference works designed for beginners. But by now there is plentiful help of every sort in Chinese and Japanese, and even a handful of useful tools in European languages.[29] Because, in recent decades, most students entering traditional medical schools in China cannot read the classical language, there are now annotated translations of the Yellow Emperor canon and a number of other classics into the modern vernacular. A few are by excellent scholars. There is even a fine textbook of medical classical Chinese (*yi guwen*) by Duan Yishan.[30]

A generation ago, every new book on medicine began with a reminder that Chairman Mao called the medical tradition "a great treasure house." That is not a bad description. More than 10,000 classical medical books survive. In them you can find material for every conceivable exploration.[31] I hope I have made a case for the usefulness of medicine to innovative research on philosophy, and for the accessibility of its rich resources.

UNIVERSITY OF PENNSYLVANIA
Philadelphia, Pennsylvania

ENDNOTES

1. See, for instance, Nathan Sivin, "Change and Continuity in Early Cosmology: The Great Commentary to the Book of Changes," in *Chūgoku Kodai Kagaku Shiron. Zoku [On the History of Ancient Chinese Science]* (Kyoto: Institute for Research in Humanities, 1991), vol. 2, 3–43; Nathan Sivin, "The Myth of the Naturalists," in *Medicine, Philosophy and Religion in Ancient China: Researches and Reflections* (Variorum Collected Studies Series), ed. Nathan Sivin (Aldershot: Variorum, 1995), chap. 4, 1–33; Nathan Sivin, "On the Limits of Empirical Knowledge in Chinese and Western Science," in *Medicine, Philosophy and Religion in Ancient China: Researches and Reflections*, ed. Nathan Sivin (Aldershot: Variorum, 1995), chap. 5, 165–90.
2. *Xunzi*, bk. 6, contains his "Refutation of a Dozen Masters." On argument and polemic in early philosophy, see Geoffrey Lloyd and Nathan Sivin, *The Way and the Word: Science and Medicine in Early China and Greece* (New Haven: Yale University Press, 2002), 61–69.
3. Sima Tan's exposition of the six trends is in *Shi Ji* (Beijing: Zhonghua Shuju, 1959), 130: 3288–92. The most important critical reevaluations are by Sarah Queen, "Inventories of the Past: Rethinking the 'School' Affiliation of the *Huainanzi*," *Asia Major*, series 3, vol. 14, no. 1 (2001): 51–72; and Mark Csikszentmihalyi and Michael Nylan, "Constructing Lineages and Inventing Traditions through Exemplary Figures in Early China," *T'oung Pao* 89, no. 1–3 (2003): 59–99. Csikszentmihalyi writes of the "common project" of each *jia* (see Mark Csikszentmihalyi, "Traditional Taxonomies and Revealed Texts in the Han," in *Daoist Identity: History, Lineage, and Ritual*, ed. Livia Kohn and Harold Roth [Honolulu: University of Hawaii Press, 2002], 81–101, at 89).
4. In Nathan Sivin, "Text and Experience in Classical Chinese Medicine," in *Knowledge and the Scholarly Medical Traditions*, ed. Don G. Bates (Cambridge: Cambridge University Press, 1995), 177–204. This article should have made clearer that the text-based pattern of transmission it describes became the norm beginning only in the late Warring States period.
5. Queen, "Inventories of the Past," 53.
6. *Hanfeizi Zhuzi Suoyin* (Hong Kong: Commercial Press, 2000), *pian* 50, 150, lines 16–24, written in the mid-third century, mentioned eight lineages passing down Confucius'

teaching, and four that transmitted the *Mozi*. Two and a half centuries later, only one lineage based on Mohist teachings had survived, but Confucian scholars claimed about fifty lineages based on eight texts. Four traditions of the *Laozi* survived through the first century AD, but all of them had dropped out of sight before the end of the Han period. For discussion, see Lloyd and Sivin, *The Way and the Word*, 55.

7. Michael Nylan, *The Five "Confucian" Classics* (New Haven: Yale University Press, 2001), 2 et passim.

8. The quotation comes from the title of Tang's 1974 article: Tang Lan, "Huangdi Si Jing Chu Tan [A First Inquiry into the Four Classics of the Yellow Lord]," *Wenwu* 10 (1974): 48–52.

9. Tang Lan, "Mawangdui Chutu Laozi Yi Ben Juan Qian Gu Yi Shu de Yanjiu—Jian Lun Qi yu Han Chu Ru-Fa Douzheng de Guanxi [The Lost Ancient Book Found at the Head of the *Laozi* (Text B) Unearthed at Mawangdui and Its Relation to the Struggle between the Confucians and the Legalists in Early Han]," *Kaogu* 42 (1975): 7–38. See also Tang Lan, "Huangdi Si Jing Chu Tan," 48–52.

10. Although Li Xueqin and others posted cautions early, the critical publication was by Qiu Xigui, "Mawangdui Bo Shu Laozi Yi Ben Juan Qian Gu Yishu Bing Fei Huangdi Si Jing [The Lost Books at the Head of Laozi, Version B, in the Silk Books from Mawangdui Are Not the Four Classics of the Yellow Emperor]," in *Daojia Wenhua Yanjiu [Studies in Daoist Culture]*, ed. Chen Guying (Shanghai: Shanghai Guji Chubanshe, 1993), vol. 3, 249–55. Among much other evidence, Qiu pointed out the obvious facts that only one of the four manuscripts mentions Huangdi, and that nothing in any of the four coincides with the many quotations from Huangdi books in texts before the Six Dynasties. No one has refuted his argument; but, as usual in sinology, a certain number of scholars ignore it.

11. There are now excellent translations of both books: Michael Nylan, trans., *The Canon of Supreme Mystery* (SUNY Series in Chinese Philosophy and Culture) (Albany: State University of New York Press, 1993); and John Knoblock and Jeffrey Riegel, trans., *The Annals of Lu Buwei* (Palo Alto: Stanford University Press, 2000). On points mentioned below, see the summaries in Nylan, *The Five "Confucian" Classics*; Nathan Sivin, "The Myth of the Naturalists," in *Medicine, Philosophy, and Religion in Ancient China*, chap. 4, separately paginated; and Lloyd and Sivin, *The Way and the Word*.

12. Kidder Smith and Don Wyatt, "Shao Yung and Number," in *Sung Dynasty Uses of the I Ching*, ed. Kidder Smith (Princeton: Princeton University Press, 1990), 100–135.

13. Although the author speaks in his preface of compiling this work in 12 *juan*, versions circulating before the Six Dynasties were in 10 *juan*, originally designated by the ten celestial stems. In the title, *jiayi* refers to these designations, and early sources cite them to refer to particular *juan*. See Ma Jixing, *Zhongyi Wenxianxue* (Shanghai: Shanghai Kexue Jishu Chubanshe, 1990), 89–98.

14. David Keegan demonstrates the character of the *Inner Canon*, in "Huang-Ti Nei-Ching: The Structure of the Compilation, the Significance of the Structure" (PhD dissertation, University of California, Berkeley, 1988). There are a great many extant Yellow Emperor texts that philosophers have not studied. The Ming *Daoist Canon [Zhengtong Dao Zang]*, reprint (Taipei: Yee Wen Book Co., 1977), lists more than thirty titles that include "Huangdi." Only the three that I discuss are of Han provenance. See Kristofer Schipper, *Concordance du Tao-tsang. Titres et ouvrages* (Publications, 102) (Paris: École Française d'Extrême-orient, 1975); and Kristofer Schipper and Franciscus Verellen, eds., *The Taoist Canon: A Historical Companion to the Daozang*, 3 vols. (Chicago: University of Chicago Press, 2004).

15. "Su Wen," in *Huangdi Nei Jing Zhangju Suoyin*, ed. Ren Yingqiu (Beijing: Renmin Weisheng Chubanshe, 1986), 8: 1–2. The text translated is "Yuan Wen Shier Zang Zhi Xiang Shi, Gui Jian He Ru." For a discussion of this and other correspondences, see Lloyd and Sivin, *The Way and the Word*, 221–22.

16. E.g., see *Lun Heng*, 54 (242, 1–10), translated in Alfred Forke, *Lun-Heng. I. Philosophical Essays of Wang Ch'ung. II. Miscellaneous Essays of Wang Ch'ung*; Mitteilungen des Seminars für orientalische Sprachen, supplements 10, 14. 2 vols. (Shanghai: Kelly & Walsh, 1907–11); reprint (New York: Paragon Book Gallery, 1962), 98–99.

17. *Shi Ji*, 27: 1289; Lloyd and Sivin, *The Way and the Word*, 223.

18. See n. 3 above. See also Kidder Smith, "Sima Tan and the Invention of Daoism, Legalism, *et cetera*," *Journal of Asian Studies* 62, no. 1 (2003): 129–56. Smith's book is important, but it muddies the waters with respect to Daoism. Aihe Wang, *Cosmology and Political Culture in Early China*, Cambridge Studies in Chinese History (Cambridge: Cambridge University Press, 2000).

19. Nathan Sivin, "On the Word Taoism as a Source of Perplexity: With Special Reference to the Relations of Science and Religion in Traditional China," *History of Religions* 17 (1978): 303–30; reprinted in Nathan Sivin, *Science in Ancient China: Researches and Reflections* (Variorum Collected Studies Series) (Aldershot: Variorum, 1995), chap. 6, 164–96.

20. Cai Degui, "American Confucianism," *Journal of Chinese Philosophy* 32, no. 1 (2005): 123–38.

21. *Han Shu*, 4: 134–35.

22. This mature relationship did not occur in earlier writings, which represent transitional phases. See Lloyd and Sivin, *The Way and the Word*, Appendix.

23. In Kristofer Schipper, *Laozi Xiang'er Zhu* [The *Laozi*, with Commentary by Xianger], in *Zhengtong Daozang*, no. 1176 (see Schipper and Verellen, *The Taoist Canon*, 74–77). All modern editions of the *Mozi*, by the way, are based on the edition in the *Daoist Canon*; inclusion does not make a text Daoist in any significant sense. See Nathan Sivin, "Taoism and Science," in *Medicine, Philosophy and Religion in Ancient China: Researches and Reflections*, ed. Nathan Sivin (Aldershot: Variorum, 1995), chap. 7, 1–72; and Schipper and Verellen, *The Taoist Canon*, 55–56.

24. Maruyama Masao, *Shinkyū Igaku to Koten no Kenkyū* [*Studies in Medical Acupuncture and Moxibustion and Their Classics: Collected Essays of Maruyama Masao on Oriental Medicine*] (Osaka: Sōgensha, 1977; 2nd ed. in 1979). Ma Jixing, *Zhongyi Wenxianxue* [*The Study of Chinese Medical Literature*] (Shanghai: Shanghai Kexue Jishu Chubanshe [revised public version of an internal publication of 1982], 1990). See the discussion of the material aspect of books in Lloyd and Sivin, *The Way and the Word*, 70–73.

25. Wu Yiyi, "A Medical Line of Many Masters: A Prosopographical Study of Liu Wansu and His Disciples from the Jin to the Early Ming," *Chinese Science* 11 (1993): 36–65. Hsiung Pingchen (Xiong Bingzhen), ed., *Rang Zhengju Shuo Hua. Zhongguo Pian* (*Let the Evidence Speak [China]*), *Lishi Yu Wenhua Congshu* (Taipei: Maitian, 2001), vol. 11, 287–318. This volume includes seven essays on cases in medical records, forensic medicine, Chan Buddhism, law, divination, and *xuean*, and on the philology of the words *an* (case/desk) and *an* (examine/comment/according to). Hsiung and others are editing a book in English on the same topic but with different content. The first published collection of medical case records was c. 1535, and its Confucian counterpart c. 1600. Legal collections long predated both. The special characteristics of medical and philosophical collections suggest direct influence.

26. Liang Jun, *Zhongguo Gudai Yizheng Shi Lue* [*Outline History of Ancient Chinese Medical Administration*] (Huhehot: Neimenggu Renmin Chubanshe, 1995), 100.

27. The Yuan History includes him in its "Biographies of *Ru* scholars (*ru xue*)" as a prominent disciple of the celebrated Cheng-Zhu teacher Xu Qian (1270–1337); *Yuan Shi* (Beijing: Zhonghua Shuju, 1976), 189: 4320.

28. He Shaochu has an anthology of writings on the *Yi* and medicine by well-known physicians from c. 1150 to 1915: He Shaochu, *Gudai Ming Yi Jie Zhou Yi* [*Eminent Doctors of Ancient Times Explicate the Book of Changes*] (Beijing: Zhongguo Zhongyiyao Keji Chubanshe, 1991). Since 1989, as He explains in his preface, this has become a fashionable topic for conferences.

29. See "Solving Scientific and Medical Problems in General Research on China," a regularly updated guide to reference materials and approaches, at http://ccat.sas.upenn.edu/~nsivin/scimed.html. This bibliographic essay is designed, not for specialists, but for sinologists encountering technical problems in their work. It gives references for all the sources mentioned in this paragraph. For an up-to-date selected, annotated bibliography of works on science and medicine in Western languages, see http://ccat.sas.upenn.edu/~nsivin/nakbib.html.

30. Duan Yishan, *Yi Guwen* [*Medical Classical Chinese*] (Beijing: Renmin Weisheng Chubanshe, 2001).

31. For a catalogue of medical works in Chinese libraries see Xue Qinglu, et al., *Quanguo Zhongyi Tushu Lianhe Mulu* [*National Union Catalogue of Primary Sources for Chinese Medicine*] (Beijing: Zhongyi Guji Chubanshe, 1991).

CHINESE GLOSSARY

an (case/desk) 案

an (examine/comment/according to) 按

Ban Gu 班固

bing 病

Chen Guying 陳鼓應

Chunqiu Fan Lu 《春秋繁露》

Daojia Wenhua Yanjiu 《道家文化研究》

Dong Zhongshu 董仲舒

Duan Yishan 段逸山

fajia 法家

Gudai Ming Yi Jie Zhou Yi 《古代名医解周易》

Han Shu 《漢書》

He Shaochu 何少初

Hsiung Pingchen 熊秉真

Huangdi Bashiyi Nan Jing 《黃帝八十一難經》

Huangdi Jiayi Jing 《黃帝甲乙經》

Huangdi Nei Jing 《黃帝内經》

Huangdi Nei Jing Su Wen 《黃帝内經素問》

Huangdi Nei Jing Ling Shu 《黃帝内經靈樞》

Huangdi Nei Jing Tai Su 《黃帝内經太素》

Huangdi Si Jing 《黃帝四经》

Huangfu Mi 皇甫謐

Huang-Lao 黃老

Hua Shou 滑壽

ji 疾

jia 家

Laozi Xiang'er Zhu 《老子想爾註》

Liang Jun 梁峻

Lishi Yu Wenhua Congshu 《歷史與文化叢書》

Liu Xiang 劉向

Liu Xin 劉歆

luan 亂

Lu Buwei 呂不韋

Lun Heng 《論衡》

Lu Shi Chunqiu 《呂氏春秋》

Ma Jixing 马继兴

"Mawangdui Bo Shu Laozi Yi Ben Juan Qian Gu Yishu Bing Fei Huangdi Si Jing"
"馬王堆帛書老子乙本卷前古佚書并非黃帝四經"

"Mawangdui Chutu Laozi Yi Ben Juan Qian Gu Yi Shu de Yanjiu—Jian Lun Qi yu Han Chu Ru-Fa Douzheng de Guanxi"
"马王堆出土老子乙本卷前古佚书的研究—兼论齐与汉初儒法斗争的关系"

Mingjia 名家

Nan Jing Ben Yi 《難經本義》

qi 氣

Qian Hanshu 《前漢書》

Qiu Xigui 裘錫圭

Quanguo Zhongyi Tushu Lianhe Mulu 《全国中医图书联合目录》

Rang Zhengju Shuo Hua: Zhongguo Pian 《讓證據説話 中國篇》

ruyi 儒醫

Shi Ji 《史記》

Sima Tan 司馬談

Tai Xuan Jing 《太玄經》

Tang Lan 唐兰

Tian Guan Shu 《天官書》

Wang Chong 王充

Wenwu 《文物》

wuwei 無為

wuxing 五行

Wu Yiyi 吳以義

xuean 學案

xuepai 學派

Xue Qinglu 薛清录

Xunzi 荀子

Yang Xiong 揚雄

yian 醫案

Yi Jing 《易經》

Yi Guwen 《醫古文》

yingyangjia 陰陽家

Yi Tong Zheng Mai Quan Shu 《醫統正脈全書》

yuan wen shier zang zhi xiang shi gui jian he ru 願聞十二藏之相使貴賤何如

Zhengtong Daozang 《政統道藏》

zhi 治

Zhongguo Gudai Yizheng Shi Lue 《中国古代医政史略》

Zhongyi Wenxianxue 《中医文献学》

Zhu Zhenheng 朱震亨

WILLIAM HERFEL, DIANAH RODRIGUES, AND YIN GAO

CHINESE MEDICINE AND THE DYNAMIC CONCEPTIONS OF HEALTH AND DISEASE

In a Chinese medical clinic a patient complains to the practitioner of chronic pain in the chest. The practitioner responds with a set of questions, some seemingly irrelevant to the problem—questions about breathing difficulties, food intake, coldness in the limbs, urination, bowel movements, mood swings, and so on—occasionally stretching the patient's memory about events in the distant past. The practitioner feels the patient's pulses at three distinct points on each wrist while staring into space in deep concentration. The chest is palpated along with other areas of the patient's body, his arm, back, feet—seemingly unrelated areas to the chest. The patient is asked to stick out his tongue and the practitioner gazes at it somewhat curiously. She comments about the spots at the tip of his tongue, his pale, shiny complexion, and his slightly purple lips. The practitioner thinks, "This is a case of blood stagnation in the heart. The spleen *qi* is deficient resulting in insufficient blood." She ponders the probable causal structure of the patterns she is observing:

> This may have been aggravated by exposure during a recent cold change in the weather. Perhaps the lack of production of blood and *qi*, complicated by digestive problems, are leading to stagnation of liver *qi* creating a vicious cycle whereby the stagnation of liver *qi* contributes to heart blood stagnation leading to further spleen *qi* insufficiency.

The practitioner decides on a strategy to break the vicious cycle by dispersing *qi* and blood by delivering acupuncture to specific points on the liver, spleen, conception vessel, and pericardium meridians. The practitioner finds that this results in a rounder, smoother pulse, reflecting improved flow of blood and *qi*, and she is satisfied with the outcome of this initial treatment session.[1]

WILLIAM HERFEL, Conjoint Lecturer, School of Humanities and Social Science, The University of Newcastle. Specialties: Chinese medicine, methodology and philosophy of technology and science. E-mail: wmherfel@yahoo.com.au. DIANAH RODRIGUES, Chinese Medical Practitioner, and affiliate of the Faculty of Science, University of Technology, Sydney. Specialties: Chinese medical practice, empirical research in nonlinear effects of Chinese medicine. E-mail: drtcm@telstra.com. YIN GAO, Lecturer, School of Humanities and Social Science, The University of Newcastle. Specialties: philosophy of ecology, philosophy of science and technology, Chinese philosophy. E-mail: yin.gao@newcastle.edu.au

What is the conception of disease operating in the above narrative of a clinical encounter of Chinese medicine? As presented in the *Huangdi Neijing Suwen*,[2] a fundamental classical text of Chinese medicine, health and disease are characterized in terms of dynamics: a subject is healthy when certain patterns of flow (e.g., *qi*) are in harmony. "Harmony" in this context means that the patterns observed reveal that the elements of the system stand in the right dynamic interrelationships. Of course these relationships are themselves dynamic, such that what is the right relationship itself evolves over time. Without over-generalizing, we can identify two aspects of this harmony. First, there must be internal coherence among the flows within the body. Second, the processes that make up flows within the body must be in resonance with the flows that make up the environment. This is an emphatic statement of what it is to be healthy. Disease is defined negatively in contrast to health: it occurs when the flows are disrupted in particular ways.

We propose to articulate this notion in Western scientific terms employing some ideas from the study of complex dynamic systems. In particular, we will focus on the complex dynamic tradition arising from the study of far-from-equilibrium thermodynamics which articulates its central concepts—dissipative structure and self-organization—through a paradigm model called Bénard convection. We hope to target one impediment to Chinese medicine being accepted and adopted outside Asia: that is, Chinese medicine's distinctive conceptions of health and disease often conflict with both the received medical wisdom and the general commonsense of those more familiar with the approach of Western biomedicine. Our aim here is not to *explain* the Chinese medical conceptions of health and disease. Rather we seek a means to *communicate* these conceptions in a way that facilitates a constructive dialogue between Western biomedicine and Chinese medicine.

I. Complex Dynamics and the Philosophy of Chinese Medicine

Far-from-equilibrium thermodynamics, developed over the past four decades, has provided insights into the study of complex dynamic systems. A central concept of this study is that of the *dissipative structure*, a structure that emerges from and is maintained by energy flow, for example, a standing wave in a rapidly flowing river. The existence and maintenance of a dissipative structure depends on energy throughput, that is, the flow of energy through the system.[3] Such structures are thus far from equilibrium: remove the energy throughput (i.e., remove the water flow) and the structure (the standing wave) collapses. The patterns exhibited by a dissipative structure are *self-organized*: That is, they emerge from the system's components' response to energy flow giving rise to new constraints reconfiguring internal interrelations within the system. So long as the energy gradient is maintained, the internal dynamics of the system maintains spatial and temporal structure.[4]

In traditional Chinese cosmology objects do not simply populate the world. Instead, the world consists of interrelating processes. The processes arise and are maintained by *qi* (energy flow).[5] What in Western terms we refer to as "objects" are in Chinese terms, stabilized patterns of a flow. So the world is quite literally a dynamic system. Each entity is a process within a process, a flow within a flow, and within each entity are processes that constitute it. Nothing exists in the absence of the flow of energy.

An example can help clarify this worldview. In Chinese cosmology the world is like a river. The river flows because of the energy differential between its source and estuary. In other words, the dissipation of energy enables the characteristic features of the river to emerge. As the river flows, waves, eddies, currents, rapids, pools, etc. emerge. We identify such features, but they do not have existence independent of the river. They exist only as the result of river flow, yet they are entities in their own right. The river is the material and energetic substrate that enables the existence of such phenomena as waves and eddies. The river is a process of flow that is differentiated into various sub-processes: waves, eddies, etc. It can be compelling to view the riverbed as the *permanent* structure that gives *form* to these phenomena. However, while at any given time the riverbed plays a role, the process of flow, including such factors as the flow rate, is also crucial to determining the location, shape, and size of such features as eddies and waves. Furthermore, change and permanence are functions of time scale. For instance, over time, water flow gives rise to such processes as erosion which impact on the shape of the riverbed. Various aspects of the structure of the river are thus dynamic over different time scales. The flow of the river and the structure of the riverbed interact over time to give rise to the dynamics of the river.

Both eddy and river are parts of the same interconnected processes. Chinese cosmology is holistic in viewpoint recognizing the interconnection of energetic processes occurring in the vicinity of the earth. Of course, for some purposes it may be useful to isolate individual phenomena. But this analysis is only a useful fiction. One could model the eddy ignoring the river that sustains it. In other words, one could black-box the energy source that maintains the eddy, but this does not grant the eddy independent existence in any material sense: When the river ceases to flow, the eddy ceases to exist. Equally important is the fact that the dependence on the river does not make the eddy any less real.

In Chinese medicine, an organism is not an individual object existing independently; rather it is an identifiable pattern within the myriad of flows that constitute the world. In the parlance of the science of complex systems, organisms are dissipative structures. The flow of food-based energy through organisms is used to reconstruct their internal structures and maintain their internal processes including these same metabolic reconstruction processes themselves. When *qi* (flow) ceases life ends. Once the energy gradient is exhausted, through the process of decay, the organism rapidly returns to equilibrium with its environment. Hence there is an intimate connection between the energetic dynamics of the organism and that of its environment. While the dynamics of human bodies exhibits self-organization, it is in constant interaction with the environment from which and within which it emerges. Ancient Chinese medical tradition characterizes the organic processes of human bodies in terms of complex flow dynamics. A healthy organism exhibits harmony both in the processes that constitute it and between these processes and the processes comprising its environment. From a complex systems dynamics perspective, key passages from the *Suwen* reveal resonances between the conception of dissipative structure, and the classical Chinese conception of the human body.

1. Qi and Flow

The role of energy flow (*qi*) in stabilizing organic structure is expressed in the *Suwen*:

> Chi Po said ... the external manifestations of the roots of life may be called the establishment of *qi*, and when the *qi* stops, transformation will cease. Therefore, each kind of *qi* has its own regulator (*zhi*[7]).... (*Suwen*, chap. 70: 553)

> The Yellow Emperor said: When *qi* starts flowing, there will be life and transformation; when *qi* differentiates into different forms (supporting various organ systems), *xing*[7] emerges.... This applies to everything. (*Suwen*, chap. 70: 554)

The growth and development of living matter is driven by *qi* (i.e., energy flow). Furthermore, it is this flow that guides the self-organization of the developing organism. The sequential developmental states, which constitute the structure or "shape" of the organism, are the consequence of the movements of energy. When *qi* ceases to flow, the organism is no longer animate. And finally the entire cosmos is to be understood in terms of energy flow:

> Everything arises through intrinsic energetic processes (*hua*), and the final outcome (*ji*) is due to extrinsic energetic processes (*bian*); intrinsic and extrinsic energetic processes interact with each other, giving rise to success or failure in life. (*Suwen*, chap. 68: 504)[8]

Elsewhere the *Suwen* emphasizes the dynamic character of organic processes:

> As soon as expiration and inspiration stop, all organic processes and transformation cease; and as soon as upward and downward movements cease, all established *qi* are in risk of collapse. Therefore, birth, growth, maturity, aging, and dying are possible only with the presence of expiration and inspiration; and birth, growth, transformation, harvesting, and storage are possible only with the presence of upward and downward movements. (*Suwen*, chap. 68: 505)

Life is a system of cyclic upward and downward movements, and these movements are related to energy flow.[9] In this process of change, movements associated with the transforming effect are called *yang*, while those contributing to structure[10] are called *yin*. In chapter 5 the *Suwen* states, "Accumulating *yang* is continually becoming the heavens. Accumulating *yin* is continually becoming the earth" (*Suwen*, chap. 5: 37).[11] The passage continues,

> *Yin* is quiet and *yang* is restless; *yang* governs growth and *yin* governs nurture; *yang* governs destruction and *yin* governs storage; *yang* governs *qi* transformation, and *yin* governs shape formation. (*Suwen*, chap. 5: 37)

It is clear that in this passage *yin* and *yang* are opposing patterns of movement. *Yin* is downward; *yang* is upward. *Yin* is passive; *yang* is active. *Yin* is quiet; *yang* is restless. Ancient Chinese philosophers saw the necessity for two fundamental manifestations of dynamic pattern to describe the animation of natural systems: *yin* is the preserver; *yang* is the mover.

2. Zangfu and Wuxing, Sheng and Ke

In *Suwen* chapter 70, cited previously, Chi Po comments on *qi*, stating that "each kind of *qi* has its own regulator . . . each [system] has its subordinate (*shèng*), each [system] has its driver (*shēng*), and each [system] has a system that completes (*cheng*) it" (*Suwen*, chap. 70: 554). This passage is a discussion of *zangfu*, which means "organ system." The Chinese notion of "organ system" is not equivalent to the one denoted in Western anatomy by "organ." It is important to note that the *zangfu* is organized around function rather than structure. Hence we talk of organ *systems* in Chinese medicine, whereas in Western medicine *organs* are anatomical structures.[12]

In order to model their dynamic relationships, in the "*wuxing* tradition," the various organ systems are mapped onto the five phases (*wuxing*), as shown in Figure 1.[13]

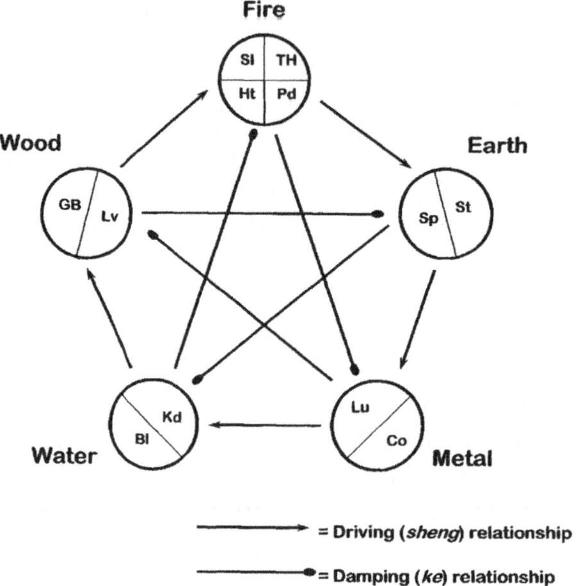

Figure 1 *Zangfu* modeled as *wuxing*. Bl = bladder, Co = colon, GB = gall bladder, Ht = heart, Kd = kidney, Lu = lung, Lv = liver, Pd = pericardium, SI = small intestine, Sp = spleen, St = stomach, TH = three heater.

In the traditional schematic representation of the *wuxing*, the phases are explicitly construed in terms of damping and driving. In terms of dynamics, *shēng* is akin to a driving force and *ke* is akin to damping force. The *shēng* relationships are driving; for instance, wood drives fire. The *ke* relationships are damping; for instance, water damps fire, in this case literally. *Shēng* and *ke* lead to periodic cycling through the five phases. Hence, the oscillations of the *wuxing* are described in terms of the interaction of both types of force.

Chapter 9 of the *Suwen* describes the interaction between the seasons, *qi* and the human body in terms of the dynamic structure of the *wuxing*. It states:

> . . . the five seasons (*wu yun*) begin; they are like a ring with neither beginning nor end. . . . The five *qi* are established in turn, and each has another that it subordinates so that it is natural for them to oscillate (*bian*) between abundance (*shèng*) and scarcity (*xu*). . . . (*Suwen*, chap. 9: 77)

Five phases cosmology describes dynamic transitions in natural phenomena. In terms of nonlinear dynamics, each organ system has its own intrinsic oscillation pattern. The organ systems are connected together as a system of coupled oscillators. The *Suwen* chapter continues with a description of an example of the interaction between the seasons and the human body:

> The Yellow Emperor asked, how does this subordinating process work?
>
> Chi-Po replied: We can calculate the arrival of [the spring seasonal *qi*] from the date of the spring equinox. If it arrives too early, then it [*qi*] is called "excessive." This results in it overpowering (*bo*) what ought not to be subordinate to it [in this circumstance] as well as overriding (*cheng*) that which is under its control. This is called *qi* excess. . . . If it arrives too late, then it [*qi*] is called "deficient." This results in what ought to be subordinate behaving inappropriately (*wang xing*), weakening that which it ought to drive, as well as overpowering that which it ought to subordinate. This is called *qi* deficiency. . . . The seasonal *qi* ought to arrive as expected, but when they are not on schedule, the five seasons are not distinct. When this happens, harmful *qi* becomes internalized, and it cannot be stopped even by a skilful physician. (*Suwen*, chap. 9: 78)[14]

This passage describes, in terms of (over)damping and (over)driving of the five-phase oscillation, how environmental factors can have a deleterious effect on the human body. If seasonal change does not occur in normal fashion, excess or deficiency of energy can cause disharmony in the organism's oscillation patterns. When the systems of the body oscillate harmoniously with the environment, and the internal oscillations within the body are harmonious, the organism is healthy. When there is disharmony, acupuncture, herbs, moxibustion, etc. can be employed to restore health. However, if the environmental disruption is so extreme that the five phases become indistinct (perhaps this is a reference to an oscillation that would be said to be "dynamically chaotic" in contemporary scientific terms), then no medical intervention can predictably restore harmony.

3. The Dynamic Perspective of Chinese Medicine

What we can observe in these passages is the articulation of a *dynamic perspective*. In the Chinese medical tradition, the human body is kept animated by the flow of *qi*, akin to the energy throughput that maintains the emergent patterns exhibited by dissipative structures. The five phrases (*wuxing*) provide an archetype of this self-organizing system, modeling the *zangfu* as a system of coupled oscillators. Dynamics is understood in terms of *damping* and *driving* forces, in much the same sense as they are in dissipative systems. The ancient Chinese believe that both the spatial and temporal aspects of complex dynamics are best analyzed in terms of damping (*ke*) and driving (*shēng*) relationships yielding *yin* and *yang* patterns *through space and time*. Thus, we can flesh out the Chinese medical notion of disease we started with. A healthy body is one in which the *zangfu* oscillates harmoniously. Disease takes the form of excess, deficiency, or stagnation in this dynamic. Such phenomena are the result of over-damping and over-driving of one or more of the fundamental oscillators in the system. Environmental factors contribute to this process. The job of the Chinese doctor is to tonify or sedate the appropriate organ system in order to restore harmony. Chinese medicine is foremost and primarily concerned with achieving and maintaining within the human body a healthy dynamic. Thus, most of the cases of ill health in Chinese medicine are cases of *dynamic disease*.

In this section, we have focused on the Chinese medical conception of human body dynamics. Nevertheless, we do not want to promote the misperception that all dissipative structures are alive. Notice that everything we have said about organisms, insofar as they are self-organized dissipative structures, applies equally to such phenomena as flames and tornadoes. Energy throughput maintains the structure of the flame and the tornado; once the energy gradient is exhausted both cease to exist. Seeing inorganic structures as animated by *qi* is present in ancient Chinese cosmology as well. Hence, while all living systems are dissipative structures, being a dissipative structure is not a sufficient condition for being alive. To make clear how the dynamics of self-organization driven by energy throughput is treated in far-from-equilibrium thermodynamics, we will articulate a canonical inorganic model of dissipative structure, Bénard convection.

II. Bénard Convection

The Bénard system consists of a shallow cylindrical vessel of fluid sitting on a source of energy as, for instance, a pot on a hot plate. The experiment starts with the fluid in the vessel at equilibrium with its environment. Macroscopically, at equilibrium, when the temperature gradient between the top and bottom is zero, the fluid is homogeneous, and it is motionless. Microscopically it is not much more interesting; the molecules of fluid pseudorandomly bump into one another. Heating the vessel from below introduces an energy gradient. The experiment proceeds by gradually increasing the energy gradient by "turning up the heat." At small temperature gradients the macroscopic picture looks pretty much the same as the initial case. But microscopically something must be happening. In general, heat rises; it does not just collect at the bottom of the pan.

At low temperature gradient the heat is transferred upward through *conduction*. The molecules near the bottom of the vessel heat up which means they start jiggling faster than they were before. If possible a heated layer would expand in all directions. In a vessel, sideward and downward expansion is constrained; thus, the heat energy is conducted upward. However, the viscosity of the fluid keeps molecules from rising perpetually. The faster jiggling layer meeting a slower jiggling layer transfers a net amount of energy into it, corresponding to a net momentum transfer; that is, the heated layer expands. The increased jiggling at the bottom is transferred up through the fluid; layer by layer the molecules begin jiggling faster throughout the fluid. Eventually, the air over the fluid is jiggling a little faster, as well. Conduction results in upward movement of heat with no net upward motion of the molecules constituting the system.

As the temperature gradient is further increased, conduction alone cannot transfer the heat up fast enough, and viscous force is overcome. Conduction becomes unstable as the hotter molecules rise faster than their kinetic energy is dissipated through viscous drag, giving them a net upward velocity. But cooler molecules above are in the way. They cannot go up as gravity holds them down, but they must get out of the way. So they sink. Randomly sinking and rising is not a very efficient way of transferring the heat upward either, so above a critical threshold of energy gradient the molecules spontaneously form traffic lanes. This organized rising and sinking is called *convection*. Since the convecting fluid, driven far from equilibrium by energy throughput, forms a stable self-organized pattern, it is an example of a dissipative structure.

The traffic lanes in the Bénard system can self-organize into variety of configurations depending on boundary conditions (e.g., the shape of the vessel). For instance, one version of the experiment takes place in a covered rectangular vessel so that the temperature gradient occurs between two plates with the fluid sandwiched in between. The common pattern observed in that case is horizontal cylindrical rolls, with adjacent rolls rotating in opposite directions like cogs in a machine. If the vessel is open to the air at the top more complex patterns are possible. One common pattern in this configuration is *Bénard cells*. This is a fairly uniform pattern of hexagonal rolls that look like a honeycomb when viewed from above. Figure 2a provides a bird's eye view of the Bénard structure.

In this structure energy throughput is achieved via the upward and downward movement of the molecules constituting the fluid (Fig. 2b). The fluid rises in the center of the cells and descends at the edges.

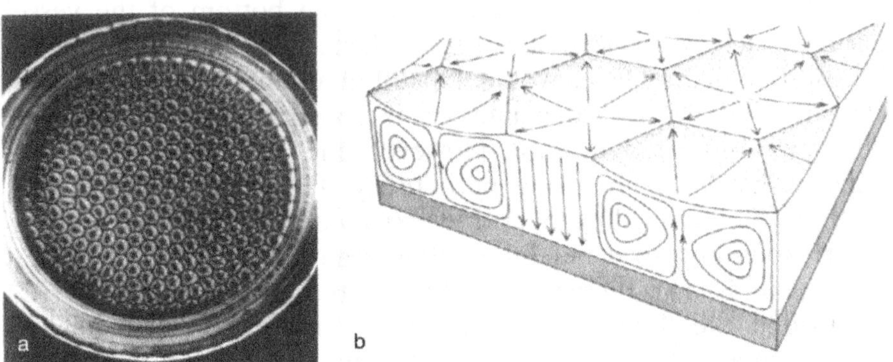

Figure 2 Bénard convection. (a) Bird's eye view showing cell structure. Reprinted by permission of Cambridge University Press.[41] (b) Schematic view showing pattern of flow. Reprinted by permission of Alan D. Iselin.

Bénard convection is maintained by energy throughput; in other words, it is a *dissipative structure*. The flow of energy through such structures gives rise to self-organized spatial and temporal patterns. In the Bénard system the pattern of hexagonal cells is maintained by the energy gradient driving the system. Although an external source of energy is required for the emergence and maintenance of some pattern of dissipation, the cellular structure that emerges is a spontaneous response of the system itself to the energy gradient. Once formed, the convection pattern constrains the flow of the molecules. Thus, the pattern exhibited is self-organized. The same idea is present in the Chinese medical characterization of the human body. *Qi* (energy *flow*) is necessary for life. However, the patterns of *qi* emerging within the body are distinct in dynamic pattern from other types of flow in the environment. In other words, the integrity of *qi* flow dynamics an organism exhibits is the result of complex interrelationships between both internal and external factors. Chinese medicine chronicles in great detail spatial and temporal patterns of *qi*.[15]

The patterns exhibited in convection are due to deterministic as well as stochastic factors. The onset of convection occurs as a precise threshold of temperature gradient is crossed in repeated experiments with a particular configuration. The critical value can be predicted analytically from deterministic dynamic laws.[16] Details of what happens after the onset of instability are not generally predictable and are held to be a function of chance microscopic fluctuation.[17] Such aspects of the patterns are *path-dependent*; that is, the particular structure emerging is a function of microscopic details of the past trajectory of the system. This introduces an historical component to the dynamics of dissipative structures. Random events in the history of the system become *locked in* constraining the future dynamics.

For example, while the global hexagonal pattern exhibited by Bénard convection recurs over repeated performances of the experiment, the local details of the pattern exhibited vary. Close inspection of a convecting fluid reveals departures from a perfectly symmetrical hexagonal lattice (Fig. 2a). Where in particular these departures occur will vary over instantiations of the experiment. They are a function of contingencies at the onset of convection. Once the cells form, however, the structure becomes locked in, and the structure changes only with severe external perturbation, for instance, shaking the vessel or removing then restoring the heat. The situation is the same, albeit much more complex, in Chinese medicine. The dynamic patterns exhibited by all human beings fit into the *wuxing* structure. Nevertheless, individuals will display idiosyncrasies in flow pattern depending on the history of their development.

Self-organized systems exhibit patterns that are the result of the interaction of driving and damping forces. In the Bénard system the driving force is the energy gradient. The damping forces include gravity and the viscosity of the fluid. It is through the interaction of these forces that self-organized spatiotemporal patterns emerge. In Chinese medicine driving (*shēng*) and damping (*ke*) forces regulate dynamic patterns. Both healthy and pathological conditions are characterized in terms of driving and damping interactions among the organ systems (*zangfu*) of the body. The five phases (*wuxing*) structure models these dynamics.

Bénard convection is a "model" of self-organization in the sense that it is a relatively simple well-understood exemplar of the spontaneous emergence of complex structure in a system driven by energy throughput. Nevertheless, the Bénard system exhibits many properties shared by more complex examples of dissipative structures. It emerges from and is sustained by energy flow; its dynamics has a historical dimension exhibiting both deterministic and stochastic elements; its structure is the result of the interaction of driving and damping forces. These features are relevant to understanding the complex dynamics exhibited by the human body. Next we will compare the Chinese medical explanations of disease with those operating in Western biomedicine.

III. Where Does Dynamical Disease Fit into Orthodox Western Biomedicine?

A dynamic approach to disease is currently emerging in Western biomedicine.[18] Applying mathematical models from complex dynamics and chaos theory emphasize the widespread significance of disease dynamics. As Canadian physiologists Leon Glass and Michael Mackey state:

> The normal individual displays a complex mosaic of rhythms in the various body systems. These rhythms rarely display absolute periodicity. . . . Whether or not one interprets normal dynamics as chaos or some other type of dynamical behavior, it is clear that many pathologies are readily identifiable by abnormal rhythmicities.[19]

If we replace "many pathologies" with "nearly all pathology" in the above passage, we would have an elegant statement of the conception of disease operating in the *Suwen* articulated in the terms of contemporary science. Although the complex dynamics approach has blossomed in a major research program, it is by no means considered mainstream.

What is the orthodox explanation of disease in Western biomedicine? This question is addressed in Paul Thagard's aptly titled *How Scientists Explain Disease*. In this book, Thagard presents a hierarchy of disease categories (Fig. 3).[20] On his account explaining disease is achieved by classification; that is, placing it into the appropriate category. For instance, influenza is a species of viral infections, which is one type of infectious disease.

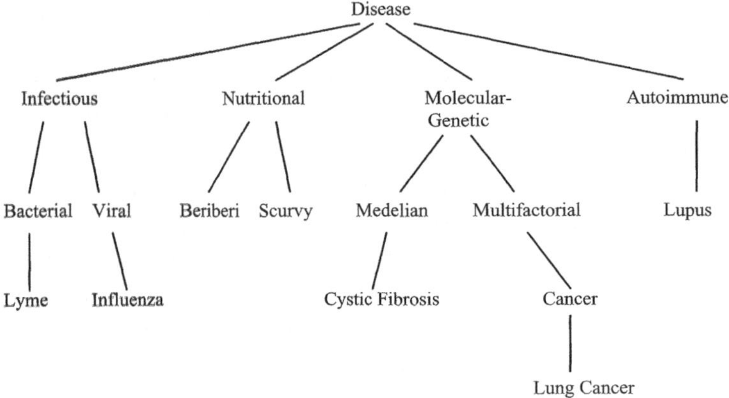

Figure 3 How scientists explain disease. Reproduced by permission of Princeton University Press.[42]

"Dynamical disease" does not appear as one of the categories of Thagard's hierarchy. This is understandable as dynamical disease is not a separate category of disease. Disease dynamics transcends the categories in Thagard's hierarchy: diseases in all categories have their dynamics. For instance, influenza is quite a complex process. The spread of virus within the infected body follows certain patterns. The immune response follows certain patterns. The various manifestations of the disease, in terms of signs and symptoms, will have patterns at both the macroscopic and microscopic (physiological) levels. In principle, these processes could all be studied *dynamically*. Nevertheless, Thagard's account ignores dynamics of disease altogether. This omission impedes understanding of the Chinese medical approach to disease in Western biomedical terms.

In an article published in 2003, Thagard and Zhu apply Thagard's model of disease explanation to Chinese medicine. They assess the discussion of Porkert and Unschuld, regarding the *wuxing* as "transformational phases" or "phases of change."[21] They recognize that,

> the five *xings* are five basic categories that can be used to classify things according to their properties and relationships to other things. Furthermore, they acknowledge that the five *xings* are not independent of each other, but have significant relationships and laws of transformation among them.[22]

However, they fail to grasp that *wuxing* constitutes a taxonomy of dynamic relationships. In the case of the human body, the *wuxing*, and specifically the *zangfu* system which is mapped onto it, models a system of coupled oscillators, together with the structure of the damping and driving relationships that give rise to system's dynamic patterns. They understand these comparisons between the *wuxing* and the *zangfu* system as mere analogies, and they reject the possibility that there are legitimate accounts of causation in Chinese medicine:

> Thus traditional Chinese medicine is closer to pre-scientific assumptions of homeopathic magic, which employs the principle that like corresponds to like, than it is to modern conceptions of causality. Thagard describes how much pre-scientific and pseudoscientific thinking is based on resemblance rather than causality. The causal mode of explanation found in current scientific medicine has no room for explanations based on resemblance and mystical correspondences, so it is difficult to compare the two kinds of explanation head to head.[23]

From our perspective, the ancient tradition of Chinese medicine provides a sophisticated articulation of the dynamics of human health and disease. It is not that the kidneys resemble water and the heart resembles fire. It is that the *dynamic relationships* between the kidneys and the heart are like the *dynamic relationships* between water and fire. This sort of analogical reasoning plays a crucial role in scientific model building. In fact, in the Western scientific study of dynamics such comparisons, even quantitative comparisons, can indeed be made. The ancient Chinese did not necessarily express these relationships in terms of causality. However, while the relationship between, for instance, *fire* and the *heart* is not causal, the ancient Chinese would not deny a causal relationship between, for instance, *water* and *fire*. Surely they would recognize that when one pours water on a fire the water *causes* the fire to be put out. But this sort of causal reasoning is too crude for Chinese medicine. No Chinese doctor wants to put out the fire in the heart! The issue here is one of subtle manipulation of complex dynamic patterns. When the heart has too much fire, one strategy is to add some water, not to obliterate the fire, but merely to dampen it, attempting to bring the system into harmony. The *zangfu*, as modeled by the *wuxing*, is a system of coupled oscillators. The job of the Chinese doctor is to harmonize the oscillations of this system through a range of strategies of tonification and sedation.

In the West the tradition of rational dynamics since at least the time of Galileo has been mathematical. This tradition eventually led in the first half of the twentieth century to the mathematical treatment of systems of coupled oscillators in the work of Van der Pol who even proposed, in an article coauthored by Van der Mark, adopting his methods to construct a coupled oscillator model of the heartbeat.[24] Since then, a range of techniques from this tradition have been applied to analyzing physiological dynamics, and this gave rise to the notion of dynamic disease. For many reasons the ancient Chinese failed to take the mathematical route. Nevertheless, their aim was to describe, classify, and analyze the dynamics of the human body. This was not predominantly a theoretic enterprise, however. Their aim was mainly practical. While inevitably Thagard and Zhu see a resemblance with "homeopathic magic," the practices of a Chinese doctor performing acupuncture are as in touch with material reality as those of a highly skilled technician tuning a complex electronic circuit by tweaking a potentiometer.

Thagard and Zhu point to the National Institutes of Health (NIH) Consensus Development Conference held in November 1997[25] as an example of successful scientific evaluation of Chinese medicine. They allow for dialogue between Western and Chinese medicine, but they hold Western medicine as the structural framework within which Chinese medicinal approaches and paradigms are analyzed. They state:

In a head-to-head clash between Western and traditional Chinese medicine, it would be necessary to choose one of the conceptual-explanatory systems as superior and reject the other. A skeptical Western physician, for example, could argue that Western medicine has incontrovertible successes and that the whole Chinese system can be dispensed with. There is no reason, however, why evaluation of traditional Chinese medicine needs to be this holistic. Some pre-scientific medical practices, such as the North American aboriginals chewing salicin-containing willow bark to relieve pain, have turned out to be medically effective even by modern standards. It is entirely possible, therefore, that some traditional Chinese therapies such as acupuncture and herbal remedies might have some efficacy.[26]

Certainly it is possible to gather evidence "proving" particular Chinese medicines and techniques efficacious according to "modern standards." There is a long tradition of subjecting such treatments to the rigors of Western science, mostly in the form of testing standardized protocols prescribed for Western-defined maladies through randomized controlled trials. There is no doubt that such work contributes to the legitimization of Chinese medicine in Western scientific terms. The point rather is that there is no compromise in Thagard and Zhu's view about the relative status of the two approaches: if Chinese medicine is to be legitimized, it must fall in line with "modern [Western] standards." There is no suggestion that perhaps the paradigms in Western medicine could benefit from some of the insights in Chinese medicine. This is indicative of how much the paradigm of Western biomedicine dominates that of Chinese medicine in scientific research.[27] Thagard and Zhu state, "The panel reached its conclusions using the standards of Western medicine."[28] This is exactly our point. Nor will mere generosity relieve the problem. As Thagard and Zhu point out the consensus panel generously "decided not to insist on the highest standards of medical efficacy based only on rigorously controlled experiments, but rather to evaluate acupuncture based on the more usual clinical standards of Western medicine."[29] According to them, the reason for this is the familiar difficulties involved in constructing randomized controlled placebo trials for Chinese medicine.

One of the difficulties they fail to enumerate is that it is fundamental to the practice of Chinese medicine that every treatment be tailor-made. Chinese medical practitioners believe that although they may recognize a particular case as an instance of an identifiable syndrome, each case is idiosyncratic, and hence the treatment must be adjusted to suit the individual. Furthermore, as the circumstances change from visit to visit—the patient may respond to prior treatment, the pattern may change on its own accord, or even the weather may change—the treatment must be altered.

According to the philosophical framework that underpins Chinese medicine, it is not that Chinese medicine is lacking in standardization when compared with Western biomedicine. Rather, from the perspective of Chinese medicine, attempts to standardize symptoms, diagnoses, and treatments are simplistic. For instance, the interdependence between an organism and its environment is not an extrinsic connection; organisms are in part *constituted* by their environment. To a Chinese doctor this means that blindly applying a standardized treatment when environmental conditions have changed is naïve.

Furthermore, understanding *wuxing* as describing a system of coupled oscillators can help us make sense of another common difficulty scientifically minded people have in coming to grips with Chinese medicine, the perceived lack of consensus in treatment strategies when one patient presents the same case to several practitioners. Originating in the articulation of traditional practice and theory, *wuxing* plays a central role in diagnostic and treatment schemas of contemporary Chinese medical practice. When we realize that what each practitioner is trying to achieve is a subtle balance in a complex dynamic system, the existence of diverse strategies makes perfect sense. Assume, for instance, they all perceive a deficiency in say the earth oscillator.[30] This could be rectified, just to identify a few obvious strategies (Fig. 1), by directly tonifying earth, and/or sedating wood (which damps earth) or by tonifying fire (which drives earth). Some strategies may be preferred to others due to details of the particular case. Nevertheless, some combination of theory, experience, and the details of the case rarely unequivocally dictate a particular strategy. Nor should they. A variety of strategies can be employed to "tune" a system of coupled oscillators. Chinese medicine accepts—in fact, embraces—this pluralistic response to complex dynamics.

However, the "gold standard" of Western evidence-based medicine is the randomized controlled trial, and such testing requires standardization in order to enable both replication and statistical analysis.[31] On the evidence-based medical model, an *n*-of-one trial only contributes anecdotal evidence. There is no a priori reason to discount the remedies of practitioners in the Chinese medical tradition. This is not to say that therefore Chinese medicine cannot be evidence-based or empirically testable. In fact, it may be possible to gather empirical evidence for the consequences of these beliefs. However, if we take the practice of Chinese medicine seriously, then we must alter medical research's presumptions about what constitutes the best scientific methods.[32] This can only be done when the beliefs of traditional practitioners are investigated as respectfully and carefully on their own terms—across cases, practitioners, remedies and through time—as are those of Western biomedical researchers.

While making the scientific testing of Chinese medicine fair, insofar as the fundamental tenets of Chinese medical practice must be respected, is a significant consideration, there is a more important reason to pay attention to the details of Chinese medical practice when subjecting it to rigorous examination. If what we have argued in this article is true, then Chinese medicine defines disease very differently than does the mainstream of Western biomedicine. Furthermore, the dynamic perspective of Chinese medicine is no less rational than the fundamental beliefs of Western biomedicine.[33] However, legitimization is only one aim of research. Far more important is furthering knowledge. It is to this issue we now turn.

IV. CONCLUSION: MAKING SENSE OF CHINESE MEDICINE

Our starting point was the uncontroversial assertion that the Chinese medical notions of health and disease are dynamic. We have shown how this conception can be effectively communicated using the framework of complex dynamics in modern science. The Chinese characterization of disease resonates with the notion of dynamic disease emerging out of recent work in biomedicine. Unlike in the biomedical tradition, the dynamic conception of disease is canonical in Chinese medical traditions.

Thagard and Zhu have addressed the issue of the incommensurability between Chinese medicine and Western biomedicine. Certainly, with its concepts of *yin* and *yang*, *qi* and *wuxing*, it is difficult to translate between the two systems.[34] We know of no one who has reconciled the significant ontological discontinuities between the traditions. This is not surprising given the vast distances of their origins. *And perhaps theoretically reconciling these differences is not the real game.* One problem with such discussions is that they are too often structured by a series of dichotomies. On one hand we have "Western biomedicine," on the other hand we have "Chinese medicine." On one hand we have "evidence based medicine," on the other hand we have "homeopathic magic." On one hand we have "modern science," on the other hand we have "pre-scientific and pseudoscientific thinking." Neither Western biomedicine nor Chinese medicine is a complete body of thought. Nor are they monoliths.[35] Both are in the process of evolution and development. So too, constructing commensurability is a process. But this process is not facilitated by the pretense that the knowledge and methods of one practice sit in a privileged position to pass judgment on the other.

What we can note here, though, is at a deep level that there is a resonance between the ancient Chinese medical tradition and contemporary research into dynamic disease. Both groups are attempting to understand the complex dynamic processes at the root of health and disease. What is necessary if Western science wants to learn from the ancient Chinese is for practitioners of Western science to have a serious dialogue with the inheritors of the Chinese tradition. A crucial element of that discussion is that it should take place in a space that is free from hegemony.[36]

A contemporary anatomy and physiology textbook discusses health and disease in terms of homeostasis:

> As long as the various body processes remain within normal physiological limits, body cells function efficiently, homeostasis is maintained, and the organism is healthy. When one or more components of the body lose their ability to contribute to homeostasis, however, body processes do not function efficiently. If the homeostatic imbalance is moderate, disease may result; if it is severe, death may result.[37]

It defines disease in terms of "a pathological process with a definite set of characteristics in which part or all of the body is not carrying on its normal functions."[38] This reflects a fundamental trait of the Western tradition: health is characterized by stasis; departure from stasis is pathological.

As the readers of this journal will be well aware, from ancient times the Chinese tradition has been obsessed with *change*. So it is not surprising that the Chinese medical definition of health is in terms of *dynamics*. Furthermore, Chinese medical treatment does not focus on *restoring stasis* but *achieving dynamic harmony*. From this perspective, very different from the Western tradition, arose a unique approach to medicine. However, the outcome parameters examined in biomedical clinical trials typically lack a dynamic component. In order to properly evaluate Chinese medicine we must understand the dynamic parameters that Chinese practitioners manipulate.

Some Chinese medical treatments have proven efficacious in Western terms. Perhaps the most stunning example is a study published in the *Journal of the American Medical Association* on the efficacy of moxibustion of "Bladder 67" for breech presentation. The treatment involved self-administered burning of a preparation of the mugwort herb (moxibustion) near an acupuncture point on the outside of the little toe (Bladder 67). In a trial of 260 subjects diagnosed with breech presentation in week 33 randomized into two groups, Cardini and Huang present evidence that, by week 35, 75.4

percent of the treatment group, while only 47.7 percent of the control group receiving only routine care, presented cephalic.[39]

Breech presentation is a handy outcome parameter for a clinical trial. Neither Western nor Chinese medical personnel would dispute its importance as a medical condition, and both traditions agree on how to define breech and cephalic presentation. However, most Chinese medical conditions do not have such tidy Western equivalents. They involve achieving harmony in bodily function described in terms that Western medicine fails to recognize. How does Western science evaluate the efficacy of Chinese treatments for such conditions?

Furthermore, assume that we accept the evidence for the efficacy of treatments like acupuncture, moxibustion, and *tuina* (Chinese acupoint massage). While there is empirical evidence, there is currently no scientific explanation for the mechanism of such treatments. However these techniques work, according to Chinese medical theory, they must involve subtle and complex processes. The best chance for revealing such a mechanism is through a complex dynamics approach. Thus, new biological processes may be revealed through better comprehension of Chinese medicine.[40]

A complex dynamics approach will bring about a more subtle understanding of causes of disease. For instance, over the past century, our understanding of infectious disease has been dominated by the "germ theory." No one would deny that *Treponema pallidum* plays a crucial causal role in syphilis. And no one would question the efficacy of its treatment with penicillin. The development of antibiotics has been a benefit of adherence to the germ theory. Nevertheless, equally undeniable is the "side effect" of the antibiotic approach in the form of antibiotic resistant strains of bacteria. Human beings harbor ecosystems of microbes, some helpful, others harmful. From the perspective of dynamics, the cause is not the presence of the offending bacterium, but dynamic disharmony. Relatively few people who are exposed to a particular strain of microbe are stricken with the disease the microbe causes. For instance, meningococcal bacteria are ubiquitous, many healthy individuals are carriers, yet fortunately few contract deadly meningococcal meningitis or septicemia. Since Chinese medicine has had a long tradition of treating diseases in terms of their dynamics, it emphasizes restoring harmony to the organism improving its ability to heal itself. This approach is particularly effective for preventative medicine. Subtle dynamic disharmonies can be detected and addressed before they manifest in disease as defined in terms of Western medicine. Perhaps this approach can shed light on the dynamic basis of disease yielding even more powerful ways to prevent and cure disease with fewer side effects.

A real strength of Chinese medicine is its dynamic orientation. It is through adoption of the complex dynamics approach that we will come to scientifically understand the therapeutic aims, effects, and mechanisms of Chinese medicine. We believe that it is through the complex dynamics approach that a fruitful dialogue between Chinese medicine and Western biomedicine will occur. Thus, our excursion into the dynamic conception of disease in the Chinese medical tradition is not merely academic: we believe that there will be important practical consequences as well.

THE UNIVERSITY OF NEWCASTLE
Callaghan, Australia

THE UNIVERSITY OF TECHNOLOGY
Sydney, Australia

THE UNIVERSITY OF NEWCASTLE
Callaghan, Australia

Endnotes

We would like to acknowledge the many colleagues who have supported this work. Professor Chuck Dyke, Drs. Rey Tiquia, Wayne Christensen, Rachael Ankeny, and Thomas Brinsmead have provided both encouragement and conversation on these topics over several years. Professor Judith Farquhar provided constructive criticism when we presented early drafts of this material at University of North Carolina in 2000. Professor Nathan Sivin provided useful comments when we presented this material at the ISCP Conference held at Sydney in July 2005. Professor Cliff Hooker and Dr. Karyn Lai have both read the manuscript and made numerous helpful comments. Dianah Rodrigues would like to acknowledge her indebtedness to Ross Penman, her mentor in the practice of Chinese medicine. William Herfel would like to acknowledge the significant impact Professor Henry Rosemont, Jr. has had in shaping his ideas on Chinese culture and thinking.

1. This narrative of a clinical encounter in Chinese medicine is fictitious. It is based on a standard case of "Heart Congealed Blood," based on the clinical experience of one of the authors (Dianah Rodrigues). The exposition of the case is somewhat simplified compared with an actual case study so that a general audience can grasp it; however, it gives some flavor of the sort of reasoning that goes through a practitioner's mind.

2. All translations from *Huangdi Neijing Suwen* (hereinafter referred to as the *Suwen*) are our own; page numbers in parentheses refer to Nanjing Chinese Medicine College Classics Group, ed., *Huangdi Neijing Suwen Yi Shi* [*The Yellow Emperor's Inner Canon Plain Questions: With Translation into Modern Chinese and Interpretation*] (Shanghai: Shanghai Science and Technology Publishing House, 1997). We have also consulted Henry C. Lu, trans., *A Complete Translation of the Yellow Emperor's Classic of Internal Medicine and the Difficult Classic* (Vancouver: The Academy of Oriental Heritage, 1978).

3. Technically, two variables are relevant to energy flow. First is the quantity of energy. Second is how ordered the energy is. The former is measured in units of energy; the latter is measured in units of entropy. Entropy is a measure of the amount of relative disorder of the energy, that is, energy with higher entropy is more disordered. Negentropy is simply the opposite of entropy. The second law of thermodynamics states that in any system with active internal energy transformations, like living organisms, entropy will spontaneously increase in the absence of energy flow, dissipating its

orderedness. From a thermodynamic perspective, for a system to increase and maintain organization it must *extract* negentropy from its environment. In the process the input energy has lower entropy than the output energy; this allows entropy internal to the system to decrease even while the overall entropy of the system and its environment increases. In the absence of energy flow system entropy would spontaneously increase. Thus, energy flow is necessary for a dissipative structure to maintain or increase internal order.

4. A good account of self-organization in dissipative structures, including the Bénard example, is found in Gregoire Nicolis, "Physics of Far-from-Equilibrium Systems and Self-Organisation," in *The New Physics*, ed. Paul Davies (Cambridge: Cambridge University Press, 1989), 316–47.

5. *Qi* is the Chinese term for energy flow, or perhaps more precisely, energy and material flow. *Qi* sustains the material structure of life, and it refers to the whole range of different forms of energy and nutrition, ranging from air to food and drink. The idea of "flow" is often contained in the term "*qi*." Thus, "*qi*" can denote either "energy" or "energy flow," and there would be some redundancy in the rendering "*qi* flow"; however, we sometimes employ "*qi* (flow)" in our article when it is important to emphasize this aspect of *qi*.

6. *Zhi* is difficult to translate. It refers to form and regularity as well as the characteristics of a process or a system.

7. *Xing* is the dissipative structure in all life. It emerges when constant energy and material flow is established and stabilized.

8. On *bian* and *hua* see Elizabeth Hsu, *The Transmission of Chinese Medicine* (New York: Cambridge University Press, 1999), 113.

9. We say "related" since the direction of causality is not clear from the passage. We are neither surprised nor bothered by the lack of specificity here. Such causal relationships are quite subtle in complex systems. In fact, (positive and negative) feedback loops are generic in such systems, thus the causal structure is often "circular." More important than identifying specific cause and effect relationships in such systems is determining the dynamic structure. This point will become important in our discussion of Thagard and Zhu below.

10. Manfred Porkert refers to such *yin* processes as "structive" in *The Theoretical Foundations of Chinese Medicine* (Cambridge: MIT Press, 1974), 19.

11. This passage, "*Ji yang wei tian, ji yin wei di*," could be more conventionally translated as "*Yang* energy continually moves upward toward the heavens, and *yin* energy continually moves downward toward the earth." However, this translation objectifies "energy," "heaven," and "earth." In Chinese ontology these are processes within processes rather than statically defined objects. Hence, *yin* and *yang* are here understood as downward movement and upward movement, respectively. A translation emphasizing this process would read something like "upward movement *is yang* energy. . . ." Thus, the heavens are a process that is formed by upward movement (which is *yang* energy).

12. *Zang*, encompassing the liver, heart, spleen, lungs, and kidneys, is translated as the "five *yin* organ systems." *Fu*, that is, the stomach, large and small intestines, gall bladder, bladder, and the triple burner are translated the "six *yang* organ systems." See discussion in Porkert, *Theoretical Foundations of Chinese Medicine*, and Nathan Sivin, *Traditional Medicine in Contemporary China* (Ann Arbor: University of Michigan Press, 1987).

13. We follow John S. Major in rendering *wuxing* as "five phases," in his "The Five Phases, Magic Squares and Semantic Cosmography," in *Explorations in Early Chinese Cosmology*, ed. Henry Rosemont, Jr., American Academy of Religion Studies L, no. 2 (Chico: Scholars Press, 1984), 133–66. See also Angus C. Graham, *Disputers of the Tao: Philosophical Argument in Ancient China* (La Salle: Open Court, 1989), 325–30. For a good discussion of the evolution of the meaning of the term through early Chinese history see John S. Major, "Substance, Process, Phase: *Wuxing* in the *Huainanzi*," in *Chinese Texts and Philosophical Contexts: Essays dedicated to Angus Graham*, ed. Henry Rosemont, Jr. (La Salle: Open Court, 1991), 67–78.

14. The five phases form a close-looped sequence with a specific order and specific relationships. There are two ways in which the five phases are related. The first is the driving (*shēng*) relationship (i.e., wood drives fire, fire drives earth, earth drives metal, metal drives water, water drives wood), and the second the damping (*ke*) relationship (wood damps earth, earth damps water, water damps fire, fire damps metal, metal damps wood). When the driving force and damping forces are in harmonious proportion to each other, the five phases follow each other with right order and pace and each phase arrives at its due time.

15. Refer, for instance, to Yin Gao, "Ecologies of Scientific Practice: An Analysis of the Organization and Dynamics of Science" (PhD dissertation, The University of Newcastle, Callaghan, NSW, Australia, 2005).

16. S. Chandrasekhar explores the standard model for the *onset* of Bénard convection in detail, in *Hydrodynamic and Hydromagnetic Stability* (Oxford: Clarendon Press, 1961).

17. See M. Velarde and C. Normande, "Convection," *Scientific American* 243, no. 1 (1980): 78–93, for a readable account.

18. This literature is becoming vast. Hobart A. Reimann (*Periodic Diseases* [Philadelphia: F.A. Davis Company, 1963]) was perhaps the first to document dynamic disease in Western biomedicine. Leon Glass and colleagues did pioneering work and published several textbook accounts including Leon Glass and Michael Mackey, *From Clocks to Chaos* (Princeton, NJ: Princeton University Press, 1988); and Daniel Kaplan and Leon Glass, *Understanding Nonlinear Dynamics* (New York: Springer-Verlag, 1995). Arthur Winfree is another pioneer of this approach who applied methods he developed in his study of circadian rhythms to heart arrhythmia (see Arthur Winfree, *The Timing of Biological Clocks* [New York: Freeman, 1987]; and Arthur Winfree, *When Time Breaks Down* [Princeton, NJ: Princeton University Press, 1987]). Ary Goldberger and his colleagues have developed a number of tools for mathematically analyzing heartbeat dynamics (see Ary L. Goldberger, "Fractal Variability versus Pathologic Periodicity: Complexity Loss and Stereotypy in Disease," *Perspectives in Biology and Medicine* 40, no. 4 [1997]: 543). Although the dynamic approach has been applied in other areas relevant to human health, those studying heart dynamics have been most prolific. See also R. M. Anderson and Ronald M. May, *Infectious Diseases of Humans: Dynamics and Control* (Oxford: Oxford University Press, 1991); Alan Garfinkel, "A Mathematics for Physiology," *American Journal of Physiology: Regulatory, Integrative and Comparative Physiology* 245, no. 4 (1983): 455–66; Richard A. Heath, *Nonlinear Dynamics: Techniques and Applications in Psychology* (Mahwah: Erlbaum, 2000); Robert Pool, "Is It Healthy to Be Chaotic?" *Science* 243, no. 4891 (1989): 604–7; and Paul E. Rapp, "Oscillations and Chaos in Cellular Metabolism and Physiological Systems," in *Chaos*, ed. Arun V. Holden (Princeton: Princeton University Press, 1986), 179–208.

19. Glass and Mackey, *From Clocks to Chaos*, 172.

20. Paul Thagard, *How Scientists Explain Disease* (Princeton: Princeton University Press, 1999), 35.

21. Paul Thagard and Jing Zhu, "Acupuncture, Incommensurability, and Conceptual Change," in *Intentional Conceptual Change*, ed. Gale M. Sinatra and Paul R. Pintrich (Mahwah: Erlbaum, 2003), 85.

22. Ibid., 85.

23. Ibid., 93.

24. Kaplan and Glass, *Understanding Nonlinear Dynamics*, 241.

25. NIH Consensus Development Panel on Acupuncture, "Acupuncture: NIH Consensus Conference," *JAMA* 280, no. 17 (1998): 1518–24.

26. Thagard and Zhu, "Acupuncture, Incommensurability, and Conceptual Change," 95.

27. Our numerous discussions with Rey Tiquia over the years have urged us to see this problem in terms of the hegemony of Western biomedicine over Chinese medicine. Volker Scheid articulates this theme in detail in "Orientalism Revisited: Reflections on Scholarship, Research & Professionalization," *The European Journal of Oriental Medicine* 1, no. 2 (1993): 23–31.

28. Thagard and Zhu, "Acupuncture, Incommensurability, and Conceptual Change," 96.

29. Ibid.

30. There may not necessarily be consensus at the level of diagnosis either, but this can be explained in the same way we propose explaining lack of consensus in treatment, through the various directions of damping and driving processes using the *wuxing* cycle.

31. For an enlightening discussion of the "gold standard," see Jason Grossman and Fiona J. Mackenzie, "The Randomized Controlled Trial: Gold Standard, or Merely Standard?" *Perspectives in Biology and Medicine* 48, no. 4 (2005): 516–34.

32. Alan Bensoussan et al. documents a study of irritable bowel syndrome with a protocol designed to compare standardized treatment with tailor-made treatment and with placebo in "Treatment of Irritable Bowel Syndrome with Chinese Herbal Medicine," *JAMA* 280, no. 18 (1998): 1585–89. It remains to be seen what the Western medical consensus will be on such evidence.

33. In fact we would argue, borrowing Stephen Toulmin's terminology, that both traditions presuppose ideals of natural order, which ought to be examined to provide a firmer understanding of both; see Stephen Toulmin, *Foresight and Understanding: An Enquiry into the Aims of Science* (New York: Harper, 1961).

34. Douglas Allchin, "Points East and West: Acupuncture and Comparative Philosophy of Science," *Philosophy of Science* 63, Proceedings (1996): 107–15.

35. Volker Scheid develops both of these points in "Traditional Chinese Medicine—What Are We Investigating? The Case of Menopause," *Complementary Therapies in Medicine* 15, no. 1 (2007): 54–68.

36. This may be politically impossible. However, we urge researchers interested in Chinese medicine to critically examine the view that the Western/Chinese medical hegemony is one based on the *intellectual* superiority of Western science. See Bruno Latour, *Science in Action* (Cambridge: Harvard University Press, 1987), esp. 179–213.

37. Gerard J. Tortora and Sandra R. Grabowski, *Principles of Anatomy and Physiology*, 8th ed. (New York: HarperCollins, 1996), 10.

38. Ibid.

39. Francesco Cardini and Huang Weixin, "Moxibustion for Correction of Breech Presentation: A Randomized Controlled Trial," *Journal of the American Medical Association* 280, no. 18 (1998): 1580–84.

40. To the credit of the NIH Consensus Development Panel cited by Thagard and Zhu, they acknowledge this possibility (see Thagard and Zhu, "Acupuncture, Incommensurability, and Conceptual Change," 96).

41. Nicolis, "Physics of Far-from-Equilibrium Systems and Self-Organisation," 318.

42. Thagard, *How Scientists Explain Disease*, 35.

CHINESE GLOSSARY

bian	變	sheng	生
cheng	成	wuxing	五行
fu	府	xing	形
hua	化	yang	陽
Huangdi Neijing Suwen		yin	陰
《黃帝內經素問》		zang	藏
ji	極	zangfu	藏府
ke	克	zhi	制
qi	氣		

KARYN L. LAI

UNDERSTANDING CHANGE: THE INTERDEPENDENT SELF IN ITS ENVIRONMENT

In Chinese philosophy, an individual is viewed as a being which is interdependent with others, and whose existence, beliefs, and actions are understood with reference to its broader environmental context. The notion of interdependent self is one that understands relationships as integral to the self: relationships with others impact on the identity of the self, as well as its intentions and behaviors. In other words, the self is relationally constituted, that is, one that is formed or shaped in part by its relationships with others.

The idea of a contextually embedded self encompasses the view that the contextual environment is a necessary dimension of the life of the individual; expressions of the self, including its actions, achievements, and value orientations, must be understood with reference to aspects of its environment. The term "environment" covers not only the natural environment but various other aspects of an individual's context, including the historical, cultural, social, and political dimensions. In Chinese philosophy, the environmental context is the locus within which an individual lives, acts, and interacts. In order fully to understand the meaning and significance of each individual's beliefs, intentions, and actions, we must have a broader appreciation of his or her contexts of operation. Chung-ying Cheng articulates this more profound conception of the environment:

> [According to a superficial sense of the term, environment means] simply "the surroundings," the physical periphery, the material conditions and the transient circumstances. . . . [However, environment] cannot be treated as an object, the material conditions, a machine tool, or a transient feature. Environment is more than the visible, more than the tangible, more than the external, more than a matter of quantified period or time or spread of space. It has a deep structure as well as a deep process, as the concept of Tao indicates.[1]

The remarks I have made so far pertain to certain characteristic features of Chinese philosophy. In this regard, I explore elements in the *Yijing* (*Book of Changes*) as it is an early text that embodies many

KARYN L. LAI, Senior Lecturer, School of History and Philosophy, University of New South Wales. Specialities: early Confucianism and Daoism, Confucian ethics, and environmental ethics. E-mail: k.lai@unsw.edu.au

of these features of Chinese philosophy (the oldest sections are believed to have been written around the ninth century BCE). In terms of the issues associated with the interdependent and contextually embedded self, the *Yijing* is an especially important text. This is because it expresses a deep awareness of the world and attends to the intricate relationships and complex causalities therein. These are primary concerns of the text, which focus on change, how it affects beings and entities, and how, as intentional beings, humans can participate in some of these processes by anticipating and responding appropriately to change.

I also intend to focus briefly on how these ideas are expressed in Confucianism and Daoism, two major traditions in Chinese philosophy, in order to provide more nuanced depth to the discussion. In both the Confucian and Daoist philosophical traditions, the self is understood in interdependent terms with others, and within a contextual environment. Passages in the Confucian and Daoist texts emphasize the importance of understanding the self in these two dimensions, as well as their implications for practical action and life more generally.

I begin with an examination of these themes in the *Yijing* in the first section before proceeding, in the second and third sections, to investigate them in a number of the early Confucian and Daoist texts. In the *Yijing* as well as the Confucian and Daoist texts, the two themes, interdependence and contextual embeddedness, are intricately intertwined. Attention to these aspects of life reflects awareness of the contingencies in life and how changes that are external to the physical self can affect it. Similarly, there is awareness of how the self, in turn, can affect others and effect changes in its surrounding environments. These issues have important ethical implications, but they also encompass more than the ethical dimension. Awareness of the interdependent self, and of one's contextual environment, also impacts on how one lives life to the utmost, as a person with meaningful relationships, and who is able and willing to contribute to and participate in the life of society. In the final section of this essay, I engage in some exploratory discussion about awareness of imminent change and how anticipation of it can be beneficial to the individual.

I. RELATIONSHIPS AND CONTEXTS IN THE *YIJING*

The *Yijing* encapsulates many aspects of Chinese thought about change that occurs within a vast cosmological framework. The text was originally used as a divination manual in the early part of the Zhou Dynasty (1122–221 BCE).[2] As a divination manual, the text has now acquired cult status among those in the contemporary Western world who are interested in alternative therapies and spirituality. However, it is not its usage in those contexts that is of philosophical interest.

From around the fourth and third centuries BCE, commentaries, known as the "ten appendices" or "wings" (*Shi Yi*), were added to the text. These appendices, together with the older hexagram sections, comprise the extant *Yijing* text.[3] The sixth and seventh chapters of the Appendices—known as the *Great Commentary (Dazhuan)* or *Commentary on the Appended Phrases (Xici Zhuan)*—are the most philosophically interesting. They are introspective in that they reflect on and explain the nature of the *Yijing* text and its applications. The commentaries attempt to articulate the underlying assumptions and rationale of divination including the interpretation of symbols, application of judgments to particular questions at hand, the explicit and implied correspondences of events across different domains (ethical, political, human, natural, and cosmic), and the scope for individual and collective human action.

In its investigation and understanding of change, the *Xici Zhuan* emphasizes the importance of being observant of the world around us (*guan*).[4] It presents a scenario, suggesting that observation was central to the derivation of the symbols of divination:

> When in ancient times Lord Bao Xi ruled the world as sovereign, he looked upward and observed [*guan*] the images in heaven and looked onward and observed [*guan*] the models that the earth provided. He observed the patterns on birds and beasts and what things were suitable for the land. Nearby, adopting them from his own person, and afar, adopting them from other things, he thereupon made the eight trigrams in order to become thoroughly conversant with the virtues inherent in the numinous[5] and the bright and to classify the myriad things in terms of their true, innate natures. (*Xici Zhuan* 2.2; trans. Lynn 1994, 77)

From his observations of things and events near and far, Lord Bao Xi is said to have acquired a comprehensive picture of the world. This passage also assumes the importance of a broader perspective rather than one that strives for specificity and definition. The aim of observation is to inform humanity about the world and, as the name of the text implies, anticipate and deal appropriately with change.

The following passages from the *Xici Zhuan* express the comprehensive vision of the *Yijing*:

> By virtue of its numinous power, it lets one know what is going to come, and by virtue of its wisdom, it becomes a repository of what has happened.... [The intelligent and perspicacious ones of antiquity] used the *Changes* to cast light on the Dao of Heaven and to probe into the conditions of the common folk. This is the numinous thing that they inaugurated in order to provide beforehand for the needs of the common folk. (1.11; trans. Lynn 1994, 64–65).

> The *Changes* is a paradigm of Heaven and Earth, and so it shows how
> one can fill in and pull together the Dao of Heaven and Earth.
> Looking up, we use it [the *Changes*] to observe the configurations of
> Heaven, and, looking down, we use it to examine the patterns of
> Earth. Thus we understand the reasons underlying what is hidden
> and what is clear. (1.4; trans. Lynn 1994, 51; translator's annotation)

While the first passage emphasizes the pervasiveness of change and
how it can affect both cosmic and human phenomena, the second
expresses continuities between these realms. In both these passages,
there is a palpable attention to the incessant processes of change that
affects all life.

The paired concepts *yin-yang*, fundamental axioms in Chinese philosophy, crystallize deeper assumptions about the ongoing transfor-
mative nature of the world. It is important to note, however, that in its
earlier usage in texts like the *Book of Poetry* (*Shijing*), *yin* and *yang*
were used only to evoke complementarity rather than change. In the
Book of Poetry, dated at around the tenth century BCE, *yin* is used in
conjunction with rain (Poem 35) while *yang* with the sun that dries the
dew (Poem 174).[6] In Poem 250, *yin* and *yang* are again used in complementary fashion, to denote the shady and sunny sides of a mountain
and to capture the regular succession of shade and sunlight according
to the position of the sun.[7] The *yinyang* polarity is not conceived of in
antithetical or antagonistic terms.[8]

Yin and *yang* are core concepts of the *Yijing*. In fact, the hexagram
lines that comprise the sixty-four symbols in the *Yijing* are called *yin*
and *yang* lines: the hexagram lines are either broken (— —), signifying *yin*, or unbroken (——), signifying *yang*. In the *Yijing*, the paired
terms *yin-yang* capture an important feature of the conceptual framework in Chinese philosophy, one that emphasizes bipolarity, harmony,
and interdependencies. The *Xici Zhuan* articulates the idea of change
with reference to *yin* and *yang*:

> In capaciousness and greatness, change corresponds to Heaven and
> Earth; in the way change achieves complete fulfillment, change cor-
> responds to the four seasons; in terms of the concepts of *yin* and *yang*,
> change corresponds to the sun and moon; and in the efficacy of its
> ease and simplicity, change corresponds to perfect virtue. (1.6; trans.
> Lynn 1994, 56)

In light of its awareness about change, the *Xici Zhuan* is emphatic
about the need to be prepared for changes in one's environment that
may affect oneself:

> The Master said: "To get into danger is a matter of thinking one's
> position secure; to become ruined is a matter of thinking one's con-
> tinuance protected; to fall into disorder is a matter of thinking one's
> order enduring. Therefore the noble man when secure does not

> forget danger, when enjoying continuance does not forget ruin, when
> maintaining order does not forget disorder. This is the way his person
> is kept secure and his state remains protected. The *Changes* say: 'This
> might be lost, this might be lost, so tie it to a healthy, flourishing
> mulberry.'" (2.5; trans. Lynn 1994, 83)

This passage alerts us to sources of change that are external to the
individual self, but that may nevertheless have a significant impact
on it. Because it holds these concerns, Chinese philosophy focuses
on processes, responses, and relational interactions, rather than on
events, absolute states, or individual entities, conceived of in independent and atomistic terms.[9] In the *Yijing*, the experience of changes is
consciously organized and articulated into a system of thinking about
reality and the place of the individual within a dynamic world.[10]
Therefore, it is critical for a person to understand his or her place in a
diverse environment with many interconnected dimensions. I now
turn to examine how these issues are articulated in the Confucian
tradition.

II. Relationships and Contexts in the Confucian Tradition

Confucianism attends to human relationships as a central component
of life. The Confucian *Analects*, the key text associated with Confucius
(551–479 BCE), focuses on relationships as integral to a meaningful
life. One of the key concepts in the *Analects*, *ren*, refers both to
specific relational attachment (*Analects* 1:2, 13:18, 17:21)[11] and compassion for others (*Analects* 12:22, 7:29). Mencius (385?–312? BCE), a
prominent Confucian, further developed these ideas of human development. He suggested that experience and appreciation of close
kinship ties, especially with one's parents, would gradually extend to
compassion for humanity. He uses the term *tui* (push, extend) explicitly to suggest the extension of the scope of human fellow-feeling,
from the particular to the universal:

> Treat with the reverence due to age of the elders in your own family,
> so that the elders in the families of others shall be similarly
> treated. . . . It is said in "The Book of Poetry," "His example affected
> his wife. It reached to his brothers, and his family of the State was
> governed by it."—The language shows how King Wan simply took
> this kindly heart, and exercised it towards those parties. Therefore
> the carrying out [*tui*: extension of] his kindly heart by a prince will
> suffice for the love and protection of all within the four seas.
> . . . (*Works of Mencius*, 1A.7:12)[12]

Mencius also believed that a child who appreciated and understood
her parents' love would reciprocate that concern and eventually

extend it to others (*Works of Mencius*, 7A.15).[13] In Confucianism more generally, we come across this belief articulated frequently: the familial context—and especially the parent–child relationship in the early years—is critical in helping a person understand the nature of relationships. In the ideal scenario, in a child's relations with her parents, she learns about relational distance, loyalty, obligation, trust, affect, competing demands, how to balance these expectations and negotiate successfully.[14]

How are these relational skills nurtured? Another key concept in Confucianism, *li* (behavioral propriety), captures a number of aspects of the cultivation of the self. In the *Analects*, the term *li* has several applications. In some passages, there is fastidious detail about bringing behaviors in line with *li* (*Analects* 3:17, *Analects* Bk. 10). In others, there is flexibility in dealing with the situation such that the requirement for behavioral compliance may sometimes be overridden by other considerations (*Analects* 9:3, 17:21). I have argued in detail in "*Li* in the *Analects*: Training in Moral Competence and the Question of Flexibility"[15] that the different requirements associated with *li* practice in some of the passages apply to those people who are less mature in moral development while other passages are more flexible about *li* because they accord more initiative to people who are more morally mature. For example, Confucius in *Analects* 9:3 argues that, on certain occasions, he sees it fit to modify *li* but not on others. In this passage, Confucius shows his initiative and maturity by providing reasons for cases when he does or does not modify existing *li* practices.

What this means in terms of the argument in this essay is that it presents glimpses into the dynamics of relational interaction. In being mindful of behavioral propriety, the young learner learns to acknowledge the fact of others around him (*Analects* 12:1). The passages capture the complexity of moral dilemmas in ordinary daily interactions (e.g., in *Analects* 4:18, 13:18, 17:21). One way to understand Confucian ethics is to appreciate its emphasis on understanding different obligations, loyalties, and relational distance in one's relationships with others, and to develop skills for interaction with others.[16] These insights and strategies are an integral part of Confucian self-cultivation, aimed at fostering an appreciation of relational proximity, affection, care, and concern. The loyalties and support networks that are an integral part of good relationships are instrumental in pulling individuals through difficult moments. As Confucian scholars including Tu Wei-ming,[17] Herbert Fingarette,[18] and Antonio Cua[19] have argued, a primary concern of Confucian moral cultivation is to develop the self in order that it is able meaningfully and successfully to relate with others.

While Confucianism recognizes the primacy of relationships, a more adequate account must also include its cosmic and spiritual dimensions. In *Analects* 2:4, Confucius' development culminates in his attunement to Heaven (*tian*) such that there was no inclination on his part to transgress the boundaries:

> The Master said: "From fifteen, my heart-and-mind was set upon learning; from thirty I took my stance; from forty I was no longer doubtful; from fifty I realized the propensities of *tian*; from sixty my ear was attuned; from seventy I could give my heart-and-mind free rein without overstepping the boundaries. (76–77)

A fuller understanding of this passage would involve detailed examination of *tian* across texts of the same period. Additionally, the concept occupied a central position in debates in the Confucian tradition, especially during the Han period (206 BCE–206 CE), and later on, in Neo-Confucianism.[20] While the discussions of *tian* are too complex to examine here, it helps to refer to one of its most significant aspects that is relevant to our discussion. The *Zhongyong* (*Doctrine of the Mean*), a Confucian text written during the Warring States period (*Zhanguo*: 481–221 BCE) and selected by Zhu Xi (1130–1200) as one of the *Four Books* (*Sishu*) of Confucianism, emphasizes cooperation between Heaven (*tian*), earth (*di*), and humanity (*ren*):

> The way of the superior man may be found, in its simple elements, in the intercourse of common men and women; but in its utmost reaches, it shines brightly through Heaven and earth.[21]

This passage expresses commitment not only to human relationships but also to the significance of human action within a broader, cosmological context. Here, the dimensions of human-relatedness and cosmological context are integrated. There is also suggestion of continuity between the different dimensions. This passage, and many others like it, have been summarily characterized by the phrase *tianren heyi*, which accentuates the cooperative unity between Heaven and humanity.[22] The phrase expresses the profundity of Confucian humanistic spirituality by highlighting the breadth and inclusiveness of ideal human action and achievement.

III. Relationships and Contexts in the Daoist Tradition

Daoist philosophy likewise holds a concept of self whose life is integrated with that of others, and whose actions and intentions are understood within a broader contextual environment. However, it is critical of the humanistic focus of Confucianism. Even if we grant that Confucian philosophy has an extensive and inclusive notion of human achievement (in partnership with Heaven and earth), the early Daoist philosophical texts, the *Daodejing* and *Zhuangzi*, are concerned about the elevation of humanity. In chapter 32, the *Daodejing* seems to propose a value-free approach epitomized by the neutrality of natural events: "Heaven and earth unite to drip sweet dew. Without the command of [humanity], it drips evenly over all."[23] The *Daodejing* rejects conventional norms and beliefs because they promote pursuit of what is strong, powerful, assertive, and so on (see, e.g., *Daodejing* 18–20). From the perspective of the *Daodejing*, a conventionally defined and guided life narrows one's perception of the others and the world:

> The five colors cause one's eyes to be blind.
> The five tones cause one's ears to be deaf.
> The five flavors cause one's palate to be spoiled . . . (121)

In contrast to conventional values that generate antagonism and strife, Daoist philosophy advocates a value orientation that is non-coercive and that allows, and perhaps encourages, more spontaneity in an individual's actions and reflections. The Daoist concept *wuwei* (non-action or non-coercive action) is frequently cited as the main concept that encapsulates a greater sense of freedom in the *Daodejing*. Although *wuwei* is applied most frequently to discussions about the approach and style of government (*Daodejing* 18, 19, 49, 60), it also refers more generally to an ethico-social framework that refrains from constraining individual and social life through the imposition of norms and conventions (*Daodejing* 28, 43, 63). Hence, *wuwei* is not merely a term that encourages passivity (non-coercion), it is also concerned *actively* with the removal of conventional boundaries to thought and action.[24] Benjamin Schwartz suggests that, in practical terms, this means that one must address the "deliberate, analytic, and goal-oriented thought and action in a plural world" (Schwartz 1985, 190).[25]

There is another important concept in Daoist philosophy that is closely correlated with *wuwei*; this is the concept *ziran*, which is literally translated as "self-so-ness." The concept connotes the spontaneous and natural response of the self to its surrounding context. In this way, *ziran* is the correlative concept of *wuwei*: While *ziran* pertains to the spontaneous articulation of the self-in-environment, *wuwei* refers to the conditions that engender *ziran*. That is, a *wuwei* approach is one that refrains from imposing conditioned responses and seeks to eradicate sociopolitical infrastructures that sustain the dominance of convention.[26]

Unfortunately, many discussions of *wuwei* do not relate it to the concept *ziran*. This is due in part to the common interpretation of *ziran* in terms of the natural environment.[27] As a result of this understanding of *ziran*, there has been a corresponding tendency to suggest that Daoist philosophy demonstrates concern for the natural environment. However, there needs to be some caution in regard to this thesis. While there are many references in the early Daoist texts to aspects of the natural environment (e.g., the *Daodejing* refers to winds, seas, rain, and the *Zhuangzi* refers to many non-human species), these references are insufficient to demonstrate that they arise from a concern to protect the environment. Daoist challenges to the status quo, including its skepticism of the humanistic orientation, might be *consistent with* concern for the natural environment. Yet, the latter may not have been a significant focus in Daoist philosophy.[28]

The concern about the restrictive nature of conventional norms and values is also shared by the authors of the *Zhuangzi*, another major Daoist text of the Warring States period. The *Zhuangzi* explores the ethical and epistemological dimensions of norms which condition the value-orientation of the people. In this regard, it is especially careful about conventional notions of wisdom which encourage superiority and argumentation (*bian*).[29] In place of conventionally valued wisdom, the *Zhuangzi* proposes a conception of wisdom that is better exemplified by examples of skilled, practical know-how that is often not expressible in words. For example, in chapter 3, "What Matters in the Nurture of Life," the expert butcher, Cook Ding—who for nineteen years has not had to sharpen his knife—is upheld as a paradigm of such wisdom (trans. Graham 2001, 63–64). Other chapters in the *Zhuangzi* whose authorship is debated, but which also advocate such practical know-how include the examples of the wheelwright Bian (chapter 13) (ibid., 139–40), the experienced ferryman (chapter 19) (ibid., 136–37), the hunchback cicada catcher (chapter 19) (ibid., 138), and the wood carver and his marvelous bell stands (chapter 19) (ibid., 135).[30]

The wisdoms exemplified by these skilled persons bring together a number of important themes in Daoist philosophy. First, they demonstrate the value of wisdom that stands in contrast to Confucian cultivated learning (see, e.g., the criticism of conventional wisdom in *Daodejing* 48). In *Zhuangzi*, chapter 13, the wheelwright Bian rather audaciously challenges Duke Huan, who is reading a book, that his knowledge is worthless:

> If I chip at a wheel too slowly, the chisel slides and does not grip; if too fast, it jams and catches in the wood. Not too slow, not too fast; I feel it in the hand and respond from the heart, the mouth cannot put it into words, there is a knack in it somewhere which I cannot convey to my son and which my son cannot learn from me. This is how through my seventy years I have grown old chipping at wheels. The

> men of old and their untransmittable message are dead. Then what
> my lord is reading is the dregs of the men of old, isn't it? (trans.
> Graham 2001, 140)

Bian's remarks suggest that the accumulation of past wisdoms is ineffectual in dealing with situations in life. Zhuangzi rejects the wisdoms from the past not because they are not applicable in any situation but because the Confucians and Mohists assumed that they were universally true or correct and applicable in *every* situation (trans. Graham 2001, 52). In contrast to the wheelwright's spontaneous judgments of how best to carve each wheel, past wisdoms are pronouncements and not adaptable to the needs of the situation. There is also a contrast between the kinds of skills that are involved; the wheelwright's in creating useful implements, and Duke Huan's in literary, word-based wisdom.[31] While the contrasts between the different models of wisdom are evident in the parable, they also prompt further reflection about meaningful pursuits in life, especially pronounced in the vocations of the two men. The wheelwright—as well as the carpenter, the butcher, and the ferryman—are engaged in the ordinary tasks of life while the Duke is primarily preoccupied with his learned wisdom. As Benjamin Schwartz notes, these skilled craftsmen in the *Zhuangzi* are experts at their tasks, engaging with the world in its ordinariness and imperfections (Schwartz 1985, 235).

Here, we should mention the context of these debates during the Warring States period. There were many solutions proposed, and doctrines debated, in addressing the sociopolitical unrest of the period. In chapter 33 of the *Zhuangzi*, the phrase *"baijia zhi xue"* referred to the author's disappointment about the narrowness and partiality of the solutions:

> The empire is in utter confusion, sagehood and excellence are not
> clarified, we do not have the one Way and Power. . . . There is an
> analogy in the ears, eyes, nose and mouth; all have something they
> illuminate but they cannot exchange their functions, just as the
> various specialties of the Hundred Schools all have their strong
> points and at times turn out useful. However, they are not inclusive,
> not comprehensive; these are men each of whom has his own little
> corner. (trans. Graham 2001, 275)

Both the *Daodejing* and the *Zhuangzi* advocate a broader outlook that transcends restricted, narrower concerns. Limitations in a perspective may occur at different levels: a person who is concerned only for his personal self-interest, or a doctrine that demonstrates interest only in human affairs. We could express this in modern terminology as the rejection of egocentric and anthropocentric perspectives. The approach in Daoist philosophy is dramatically different from a normative one that begins at the level of standardization and which interprets aberrations as deviances from the norm.

Daoist philosophy draws attention to diversity in the world.[32] From this perspective, it is important to understand connections and interdependencies in order to respond appropriately and efficaciously. Roger Ames draws on the concept *shi* to express the importance of efficacy in Zhuangzi's philosophy of action.[33] According to Ames, *shi* captures the importance of understanding the situation and grasping the moment:

> ... the Chinese notion of "situationality" is captured in *shi*, which, as an ongoing process that includes agency within it, means at once "situation," "momentum," and "manipulation." *Shi* includes all of the conditions that collaborate to produce a particular situation, including place, agencies, and actions. (Ames 1998, 227)

This feature of Daoist philosophy is also noted by a number of other scholars. Angus Graham describes Daoist wisdom in terms of "knowing how": "The Taoist art of living is a supremely intelligent responsiveness which would be undermined by analysing and choosing, and ... grasping the Way is an unverbalizable 'knowing how' rather than 'knowing that'" (trans. Graham 2001, 186).[34] In terms of thinking about the self and appropriate action, Kuang-Ming Wu argues that Zhuangzi's philosophy addresses its reader personally, as a challenge to engage in critical self-reflection. Wu contends that such self-reflection has important implications for an individual's engagement with the affairs of the world, not least because it helps to engender spontaneous efficacy in dealing with changing situations.[35] In the final section of this essay, I discuss some practical implications of a person's awareness of his susceptibility to changes in the broader, contextual environment. I consider this issue by discussing a person's preparedness for and ability to deal with change.

IV. Some Reflections on Understanding and Anticipating Change

In this section, I refer to a small number of examples from cross-cultural psychological research to help our reflections on these issues. Some researchers in cross-cultural psychology argue that there are significant differences in the way people in Asian and Western countries perceive and interpret situations, events, and relationships.[36] We must exercise caution about the many subtleties embedded in these suggestions. These studies should not neglect more specific demographic and local characteristics of people in these broad geographical groupings.[37] Additionally, much care needs to be taken to avoid essentialist conceptions of personhood that are culturally based. For example, some studies of people of Asian origin who live in Western countries, and who have spent a significant portion of their lives there, show that the responses of these people are more closely aligned with those of their counterparts in their countries of abode than with those of their cultural heritage.[38]

I refer to these empirical studies with some restraint, not wishing to suggest that elements of Chinese philosophy are necessary and sufficient for the way ethnic Chinese people understand the world and deal with situations. The research data on people in Japan and Korea reveal that they do also attend to relational and contextual factors in their experiences of the world, although there are subtler, yet significant differences across these groups of people.[39] In this essay, I do not presuppose any causal connection between Chinese philosophy and the psychology of Chinese people. The discussion of findings in cross-cultural psychology helps us to understand how cognitive conceptions of self might possibly be realized in everyday, practical contexts. In other words, they are used for illustrative purposes.

The examination of texts and themes in the preceding sections reveals attentiveness to factors that are connected with change. Such attentiveness derives from awareness of oneself as an individual in a broader relational and contextual environment, and therefore susceptible to changes that might occur in those circumstances. Of these changes, many are significant, irreducible, and not universalizable. Furthermore, the causal connections may not be explained in terms of simple causal chains. This approach stands in contrast to those with a relatively narrower focus, either on singular entities, their properties, or simple causal relations.

How might these notions of self inform practical action? If a person understands the self as constituted in part by relational and contextual factors, then she should also be mindful of changes brought about by these. Needless to say, the greater the number of variables at play, the greater the likelihood of change. From the perspective of a person who holds this view, the world is a complex place comprised by individuals and relationships that are not reducible to separate beings or units. Such a viewpoint may be captured by the metaphor of a panoramic, wide-angled lens as opposed to one that has a "zoom-in" or magnified focus on a particular aspect of the whole. The view from wide-angled lenses capture a broader scope that may include seemingly tangential factors while the view from a magnifying lens focuses on an isolated section of a larger picture. This metaphor emphasizes the major impact these lenses—perspectives—have on how one perceives, understands, and interprets the world. From the point of view of a wide-angle lens, the world is plural and diverse and, indeed, a rather complicated place.

To illustrate the differences between a more inclusive and a more focused worldview, we may refer to a study in 1998 of four- and six-year-old American, Korean, and Chinese children. These children were asked to engage in a variety of autobiographical narratives. For instance, they were asked to relate a story from pictures and report on events, such as the things they did at bedtime the night before or how they spent their last birthday. In comparison with the American children, the Chinese children provided more general detail about events and discussed them in a brief, matter-of-fact way. By contrast, American children described many fewer, specific episodes while providing almost three times as many details about each of the episodes. Although all children made more references to themselves than to others, the proportion of self-references was more than three times higher in the case of the American children.[40]

Returning to the metaphor of the different lenses, we need to note that there are some limitations in the example as it does not necessarily capture the dynamism in the worldview espoused in Chinese philosophy. The philosophy of the *Yijing* in particular focuses not only on viewing situations from a broader perspective. It also advocates the importance of understanding that life is very much characterized by both continuity and flux. The concern about change and how one can effectively respond to new situations is also present in Confucianism and Daoism, as we have seen in the preceding discussion. While Confucianism emphasizes the self as constituted in part by an individual's key relationships, Daoism highlights the self that is embedded within a particular environmental context and hence subject to the fluctuation of factors therein. Both philosophies recognize that the impact of changes can be significant and can potentially bear on the self.[41]

The belief that individuals and situations are susceptible to change will prompt one who is practically wise to prepare for change and to think about strategies to deal with change. From a prudential point of view, one does not assume that stability is the norm but instead should be prepared for contingency. This is clearly articulated in the *Yijing* passage we have previously examined, which warns that "to get into danger is a matter of thinking one's position secure . . ." (*Xici Zhuan* 2.5; trans. Lynn 1994, 83).

In a psychological study involving American and Chinese university students in relation to their attitudes to and expectations of change, the Chinese students thought change was likely about fifty percent of the time. American students thought change was likely about thirty percent of the time.[42] Summarily, the results of this particular study show that the Chinese students were (i) more likely to predict change; (ii) predicted more change; and (iii) predicted more change in the rate of change. Interestingly, some Chinese university students, when asked to reflect on change, commented that people who predicted change were deemed wise.[43]

Understanding change and knowing how to respond are important aspects of the philosophy of the *Yijing* as well as in the early Confucian and Daoist texts. A quick survey of other texts of the Spring and Autumn (*Chunqiu*) and Warring States periods would demonstrate a similar inclination. The texts include *Sunzi Bingfa* (Sunzi's *Art of War*), the *Liezi*, the *Lu Shi Chunqiu* (*Spring and Autumn Annals of Master Lu*), as well as others dealing with alchemy and human health.[44] Collectively, these texts reveal a focus on an integrated and comprehensive worldview, the connections between the different parts in the world, the relationships between entities, the complexity of causes and effects, the place of humanity in a constantly transforming world, and the importance of individual actions and responses. It is apt here to cite Angus Graham's description of Zhuangzi's *modus operandi* as a paradigmatic model of responsiveness to others and the world around:

> People who really know what they are doing, such as cooks, carpenters, swimmers, boatmen, cicada-catchers, whose instruction is always available to any philosopher or emperor who has the sense to listen to them, do not go in much for analyzing, posing alternatives, and reasoning from first principles. They no longer even bear in mind any rules they were taught as apprentices. They attend to the total situation and respond, trusting to a knack which they cannot explain in words, the hand moving of itself as the eye gazes with unflagging concentration.[45]

I suggest there are conceptual resources in Chinese philosophy that promote a wider, more inclusive perspective and that encourages its readers to think of the self in terms of its interdependencies and relationships. There is a need to explore more fully these aspects of Chinese philosophy in texts associated with the different Chinese philosophical traditions. In addition, interdisciplinary philosophical and psychological research will be particularly fruitful if it can appropriately identify some correlations between Chinese philosophical ideas and efficacious responses to change. If my thesis is correct that Chinese philosophy has resources for psychological well-being, we should be encouraging not only scholarly study but also a more widespread, general readership of its texts.

UNIVERSITY OF NEW SOUTH WALES
Sydney, Australia

ENDNOTES

I am indebted to Professor Chung-ying Cheng for his detailed and thoughtful comments on an earlier version of this essay.

1. Chung-ying Cheng, "On the Environmental Ethics of the *Tao* and the *Ch'i*," *Environmental Ethics* 8, no. 4 (1986): 351–70, at 353.
2. The original text included symbols, called "hexagrams," each comprised by six lines, broken or unbroken. Each of the sixty-four hexagrams is accompanied by statements describing the symbol as a whole (*guaci*) as well as statements on each of its lines according to their position in the hexagram (*yaoci*). In divination, yarrow stalks were cast and used to identify the correct hexagram pertaining to a particular issue, and the symbol and lines statements were interpreted to fit the circumstances. Refer to Richard John Lynn, trans., *The Classic of Changes: A New Translation of the I Ching as Interpreted by Wang Bi* (New York: Columbia University Press, 1994), 1–23. In the following text page numbers of the same book will be shown in parenthesis.
3. Traditionally, it was believed that all "Ten Wings" were believed to have been written by Confucius, although modern scholarship is not convinced this is the case. The language, material, and treatment of topics in the different appendices suggest different authorship over time. (ibid.)
4. Chung-ying Cheng states that observation is a fundamental aspect of the *Yijing*, marking it with the phrase the "observational origins of the *Yijing*," in Chung-ying Cheng, "Philosophy of Change," *Encyclopaedia of Chinese Philosophy*, ed. Antonio Cua (New York: Routledge Publishing, 2003), 517–24, at 518–19.
5. The "numinous" is Lynn's translation of the term *shen*, which has a sense of the spiritual. The *Yijing* emphasizes a person's ability to understand the numinous realm. In some cases, sages are said to have numinous power to apply the wisdom of the *Yijing* in alignment with the numinous realm of Heaven and Earth (refer to Lynn 1994, n. 11 at 70).
6. References to the *Book of Poetry* are from the translation by James Legge, *The Chinese Classics*, vol. IV, The She King, 2nd ed. with minor text corrections (Taipei: SMC Publishing, 1935).
7. Benjamin Schwartz, *The World of Thought in Ancient China* (Cambridge and London: The Belknap Press of Harvard University Press, 1985), 355. In the following text, page numbers of the same book will be provided in parenthesis.
8. John Henderson suggests that the conceptual binary framework of *yinyang* as reciprocal, interdependent, and dynamic dominated Chinese thinking, so much as to eclipse earlier conceptions of dualism in China (in John Henderson, "Cosmology," in *Encyclopaedia of Chinese Philosophy*, ed. Antonio Cua [New York: Routledge Publishing, 2003], 187–94, at 191). See also John S. Major, *Heaven and Earth in Early Han Thought: Chapters Three, Four and Five of the Huainanzi* (SUNY Series in Chinese Philosophy and Culture) (Albany: State University of New York Press, 1993), 28.
9. Chinese philosophy upholds a connected and comprehensive ontology. This comprehensive and integrated ontology underlies discussions of ethics, government, language, natural philosophy and reasoning and argumentation. Chung-ying Cheng has written extensively about ontology as the basis of many aspects of Chinese philosophy. See especially his "Dimensions of the Dao and Onto-Ethics in Light of the DDJ," *Journal of Chinese Philosophy* 31, no. 2 (2004): 143–82; and his essay in this volume "On Human Consciousness in Classical Chinese Philosophy" (at 9–32).
10. Chung-ying Cheng, "The Origins of Chinese Philosophy," in *Companion Encyclopaedia of Asian Philosophy*, ed. Brian Carr and Indira Mahalingam (London: Routledge Publishing, 1997), 493–534, at 502.
11. The translations of the *Analects* in this essay are taken from *The Analects of Confucius: A Philosophical Translation*, trans. Roger Ames and Henry Rosemont, Jr. (New York: Ballantine, 1998), unless otherwise noted.
12. From *The Four Books*, trans. James Legge (Taiwan: Culture Book Company, 1981), 456–57. All other references to the *Works of Mencius* are from Legge's translation and page numbers are shown in parenthesis.

13. He was, however, also aware of the difficulties associated with this suggestion. In the discussions in the *Works of Mencius*, he addresses the concerns of Mozi (480?–390? BCE), who argued that the Confucian emphasis on special relationships would have the opposite effect in terms of bringing about social order. According to Mozi, Confucianism advocated discrimination between kin and non-kin and therefore actively promoted partiality and division in society (see, e.g., *Mozi*, chapter 39: "Against Confucianism," in *Ethical and Political Works of Mo Tzu*, trans. Yi-pao Mei [London: Arthur Probsthain, 1929], 200). To this, Mencius replies that there should really only be one "root" (*ben*: basis) of human compassion, but that the Mohists make it two (*Works of Mencius*, 3A.5:3; trans. Legge 1981, 640–41).
14. Refer to the discussion of filial piety in Karyn Lai, *Learning from Chinese Philosophies: Ethics of Interdependent and Contextualised Self* (Aldershot: Ashgate Publishing, 2006), 25–30.
15. Karyn L. Lai, "*Li* in the *Analects*: Training in Moral Competence and the Question of Flexibility," *Philosophy East and West* 56, no. 1 (2006): 69–83.
16. I discuss this topic in Karyn L. Lai, "Confucianism as a Skills-Based Ethic," in *Learning from Chinese Philosophies: Ethics of Interdependent and Contextualised Self* (Aldershot: Ashgate Publishing, 2006), 109–24.
17. Tu Wei-ming, *Confucian Thought: Selfhood as Creative Transformation* (Albany: State University of New York Press, 1985).
18. Herbert Fingarette's relevant works on this topic include *Confucius: The Secular as Sacred* (New York: Harper and Row, 1972); "The Problem of the Self in the *Analects*," *Philosophy East and West* 29, no. 2 (1979): 129–40; and "The Music of Humanity in the *Conversations* of Confucius," *Journal of Chinese Philosophy* 10, no. 3 (1983): 331–56.
19. Antonio S. Cua is perhaps the most insightful and prolific contemporary philosopher on the topic of moral theory and ethical cultivation in Confucian thought (in English-language publications). Cua's publications in this area include "Reasonable Action and Confucian Argumentation," *Journal of Chinese Philosophy* 1, no. 1 (1973): 57–75; *Dimensions of Moral Creativity* (University Park: Pennsylvania State University Press, 1978); "Tasks of Confucian Ethics," *Journal of Chinese Philosophy* 6, no. 1 (1979): 55–67; "Confucian Vision and Human Community," *Journal of Chinese Philosophy* 11, no. 3 (1984): 227–38; "Reflections on Moral Theory and Understanding Moral Traditions," in *Interpreting Across Boundaries*, ed. Gerald Larson and Eliot Deutsch (Princeton: Princeton University Press, 1988), 280–93; "The Status of Principles in Confucian Ethics," *Journal of Chinese Philosophy* 16, nos. 3–4 (1989): 273–96; "The Conceptual Framework of Confucian Ethical Thought," *Journal of Chinese Philosophy* 23, no. 2 (1996): 153–74; "The Nature of Confucian, Ethical Tradition," *Journal of Chinese Philosophy* 23, no. 2 (1996): 133–51; and *Moral Vision and Tradition: Essays in Chinese Ethics* (Washington: Catholic University of America Press, 1998).
20. During the Han Dynasty, thinkers synthesized concepts and themes from different doctrine and schools. They also engaged in a wide range of topics, including cosmology, astronomy, politics, society and its institutions, ethics, health, and personal well-being. They drew correlations and continuities between events in many of these realms; these developments were influential in shaping Neo-Confucianism, the dominant philosophical force right through to Qing Dynasty (1644–1912) in China. Refer to Henderson, "Cosmology," 187–94. An authoritative account of the developments in the concept *tian* during the Han period is presented by Major, *Heaven and Earth in Early Han Thought*.
21. James Legge, trans., *Zhongyong*, 12:4, in *The Four Books* (Taiwan: Culture Book Company, 1981), 57.
22. Chung-ying Cheng draws together elements in Chinese philosophy that comprise the philosophy of *tianren heyi* in "On the Metaphysical Significance of *Ti* (Body-Embodiment) in Chinese Philosophy: *Benti* (Origin-Substance) and *Ti-Yong* (Substance and Function)," *Journal of Chinese Philosophy* 29, no. 2 (2002): 145–61. In his discussion, the different disciplinary fields in Western philosophy—metaphysics, epistemology, and ethics—are integrated. He discusses the notion of *benti*, metaphysical source-substance, suggesting that to know reality and its "onto-cosmological root" is

to understand life more broadly (at 155). In this way, substance and function are unified; *tianren heyi* is both a metaphysical and ethical doctrine. In relation to the argument here, for a person to understand the self more broadly is also for her to have a value-orientation toward relationships and context.

23. Unless otherwise stated, translations of the *Daodejing* are by Wing-tsit Chan, *The Way of Lao Tzu* (Upper Saddle River: Prentice Hall, The Library of Liberal Arts, 1963), 157.

24. Graham emphasizes the importance of retaining both these aspects of *wuwei*, in Angus C. Graham, *Disputers of the Tao: Philosophical Argument in Ancient China* (La Salle: Open Court, 1989), 232. Chad Hansen argues convincingly that there are broader implications of *wuwei*, given that to "*wei*" is to "deem" (Chad Hansen, *A Daoist Theory of Chinese Thought* [New York: Oxford University Press, 1992], 212–14). According to this thesis, a person who is steeped in conventional norms *deems* (*wei*) everything in conventional terms. To *wuwei* is to act in a manner that is not constrained by conventional norms and values.

25. Schwartz interprets Daoist *wuwei* as a reaction to the Mohist goal-directed activity, which is ". . . based on an accurate analytic knowledge of the factors which bear on the situation at hand and on an accurate 'weighing' of such factors" (see Schwartz, *World of Thought in Ancient China*, 190).

26. I discuss this in greater detail in Lai, *Learning from Chinese Philosophies*, 96–105.

27. This may be accounted for partly by the dominance of Wang Bi's (226–249 CE) interpretation of the *Daodejing*. His influential interpretation of the text proposes a naturalistic reading of *ziran* (*Commentary on the Lao Tzu by Wang Pi*, trans. Ariane Rump, in collaboration with Wing-tsit Chan, Monographs for the Society of Asian and Comparative Philosophy, no. 6 [Honolulu: University Press of Hawai'i, 1979]). Contemporary discussions of *ziran* in naturalistic terms have been proposed by Xiaogan Liu, "An Inquiry into the Core Value of Laozi's Philosophy," in *Religious and Philosophical Aspects of the Laozi*, ed. Mark Csikszentmihalyi and Philip Ivanhoe (Albany: State University of New York Press, 1999), 211–38; and Philip Ivanhoe, *The Daodejing of Laozi* (New York: Seven Bridges Press, 2002), 25.

28. Refer to the discussion in Karyn L. Lai, "Conceptual Foundations for Environmental Ethics: A Daoist Perspective," *Environmental Ethics* 25, no. 3 (2003): 247–66.

29. Refer to *Zhuangzi*, chapter 2, "The Sorting which Evens Things Out," where Zhuangzi describes the competition between the Confucians and Mohists (*Chuang-Tzu: The Inner Chapters*, trans. Angus C. Graham [Indianapolis: Hackett Publishing Company, 2001], 52) and his comment on arguing over alternatives (Ibid., 60). In the following, page numbers of the same book will be provided in parenthesis.

30. Angus C. Graham discusses authorship issues of the *Zhuangzi* in an authoritative discussion, "How Much of *Chuang Tzu* Did Chuang Tzu Write?" in *A Companion to Angus C. Graham's Chuang Tzu*, ed. Harold Roth, Monograph no. 20, Society for Asian and Comparative Philosophy (Honolulu: University of Hawai'i Press, 2003), 58–103; originally published in Henry Rosemont, Jr. and Benjamin Schwartz, eds., *Studies in Classical Chinese Thought*, Journal of the American Academy of Religion Thematic Studies (Chico: Scholars Press, 1980).

31. The debates during the Warring States period around the time when sections of the *Zhuangzi* are believed to have been written focused on *bian*, argumentation. These debates focused especially on semantic considerations (more specifically on the correspondences between name [*ming*] and reality [*shi*]). Refer to Graham's discussion in "How Much of *Chuang Tzu* Did Chuang Tzu Write?" (ibid.) The Later Mohists were major participants in this debate, see Christopher Fraser, "Introduction: Later Mohist Logic, Ethics, and Science after 25 Years," in *Later Mohist Logic, Ethics, and Science*, ed. A. C. Graham (Hong Kong: Chinese University Press, 2003), xvii–xxxiv.

32. For a discussion of the perspective of plurality in the *Zhuangzi*, refer to Karyn Lai, "Philosophy and Philosophical Reasoning in the *Zhuangzi*: Dealing with Plurality," *Journal of Chinese Philosophy* 33, no. 3 (2006): 365–74.

33. Roger Ames, "Knowing in the *Zhuangzi*: From Here, on the Bridge, over the River Hao," in *Wandering at East in the Zhuangzi*, ed. Roger Ames (Albany: State

University of New York Press, 1998), 219–30. In the following, page numbers of the same book will be provided in parenthesis.

34. I discuss the distinction between "great wisdom" (*dazhi*) and "little wisdom" (*xiaozhi*) of the *Zhuangzi* text, in Lai, "Philosophy and Philosophical Reasoning in the *Zhuangzi*," 373.

35. Kuang-ming Wu, *Chuang Tzu: World Philosopher at Play*, American Academy of Religion Studies in Religion, no. 26 (New York: Crossroad Publishing, 1982). See also Alan Fox, "Reflex and Reflectivity: *Wuwei* in the *Zhuangzi*," *Asian Philosophy* 6, no. 1 (1996): 59–72.

36. See, for example, Richard Nisbett, *The Geography of Thought: How Asians and Westerners Think Differently . . . and Why* (London: Nicholas Brealey Publishing, 2003); Serena Chen, Tammy English, and Kaiping Peng, "Self-Verification and Contextualized Self-Views," *Personality and Social Psychology Bulletin* 32, no. 7 (2006): 930–42; Kaiping Peng, Julie Spencer-Rodgers, and Zhong Nian, "Naïve Dialecticism and the Tao of Chinese Thought," in *Indigenous and Cultural Psychology: Understanding People in Context*, ed. Uichol Kim, Kuo-Shu Yang, and Kwang-Kuo Hwang (New York: Springer, 2006), 247–62.

37. See, for example, Dora Dien, *Confucianism and Cultural Psychology: Comparing the Chinese and Japanese* (Hayward: California State University, 1997). Refer also to the discussion in Nisbett, *The Geography of Thought*, 71–77.

38. Refer, for example, to Kaiping Peng and Eric Knowles, "Culture, Education, and the Attribution of Physical Causality," *Personality and Social Psychology Bulletin* 29, no. 10 (2003): 1272–84; Ying-yi Hong, Michael Morris, Chie-yue Chiu, and Veronica Benet-Martinez, "Multicultural Minds: A Dynamic Constructivist Approach to Culture and Cognition," *American Psychologist* 55, no. 7 (2000): 709–20; and Nisbett, *The Geography of Thought*, 226–28.

39. Refer to n. 36 and n. 37.

40. Jessica Jungsook Han, Michelle Leichtman, and Qi Wang, "Autobiographical Memory in Korean, Chinese and American Children," *Developmental Psychology* 34, no. 4 (1998): 701–13.

41. The Mohists and Legalists sought to control the nature of change and reduce its scope by advocating the imposition of standards (*fa*) that were applicable to all individuals and situations. However, *fa* in Legalist philosophy was an implement for control of the people; the ruler was not subject to it. While the Mohists' ultimate concern was to promote stability and social utility, the Legalists were concerned to control change in order to maintain the power of the ruler.

42. The students were shown graphs exhibiting some trends (upward, downward, of various curvatures) and asked to predict future trends. The American students made more predictions consistent with the trends shown in the graphs. If a particular trend went up, the Americans were more likely to predict that it would continue going up than were the Chinese. If the trend went down, the Americans were more likely to predict decline would continue than were the Chinese. The research is reported by Li-Jun Ji, Yanjie Su, and Richard Nisbett, "Culture, Change and Prediction," *Psychological Science* 12, no. 6 (2001): 450–57.

43. Ibid., 455.

44. Refer to Nathan Sivin's discussion "Philosophy of Medicine" in this volume (at 43–56).

45. A. C. Graham, "Taoist Spontaneity and the Dichotomy of 'Is' and 'Ought,'" *Experimental Essays on Chuang-tzu*, ed. Victor Mair (Honolulu: University of Hawai'i Press, 1983), 7.

CHINESE GLOSSARY

Bao Xi	包羲	bian	辯
Benti	本體	*Chunqiu*	《春秋》

dao	道	shi (actual, real)	實
Daodejing	《道德经》	shi (power, momentum)	勢
dazhi	大知	*Shijing*	《詩經》
"Dazhuan"	"大傳"	"Shi Yi"	"十翼"
di	地	*Sishu*	《四書》
fa	法	*Sunzi Bingfa*	《孫子兵法》
guaci	卦辭	tian	天
guan	觀	tui	推
Huainanzi	《淮南子》	wuwei	無為
jianai	兼爱	wuxing	五行
li	禮	xiaozhi	小知
Liezi	《列子》	"Xici Zhuan"	"系辭傳"
Lu Shi Chunqiu	《呂氏春秋》	*Yijing*	《易经》
ming	名	yinyang	陰陽
Peng	鵬	Zhanguo	戰國
ren (humaneness, benevolence)	仁	*Zhongyong*	《中庸》
		Zhuangzi	庄子
ren (human person)	人	*Zhuangzi*	《庄子》
tianren heyi	天人合一	ziran	自然

LAUREN F. PFISTER

ENVIRONMENTAL ETHICS AND SOME PROBING QUESTIONS FOR TRADITIONAL CHINESE PHILOSOPHY

As a philosopher who has lived and taught in Hong Kong for the past twenty years, being regularly involved in academic conversations and research in Mainland China during this period, I am pursuing here an exercise in self-reflective criticism and descriptive ethics. The focus of my arguments is almost always directed to the narrower circles of those with whom I myself identify, those of us who are writing and exploring Chinese philosophical issues within the realms of the Ruist ("Confucian"), Daoist, and Chinese Buddhist traditional teachings. These include not only Chinese philosophers writing in Chinese and English, but also those of us in "cultural China"[1] (*wenhua Zhongguo*) who address Chinese philosophical problems from any of these perspectives. As a result, much of what I reflect upon here, especially near the end of this essay, comes from more personal, situated, and practical perspectives about matters that have become experienced traumata in Hong Kong and Mainland China during the past two decades.

In the initial two sections of what follows I provide details about the relative lack of influence that reflects on environmental ethics by "traditional Chinese philosophers" (meaning those representing the Chinese traditional teachings mentioned above) in Anglophone scholarly circles where environmental ethics is regularly discussed. In this context I indicate briefly five theoretical issues in environmental ethics which we traditional Chinese philosophers, whether writing in English or Chinese, have not yet provided responses which other environmental ethicists who normally do not work in Chinese philosophical circles have taken up as definitive answers to these problems. That there have been some substantial contributions in this regard especially by 2005 is promising, but I will indicate why these problems remain serious and significant. Following this, in the third section I highlight a theoretical problem which became clear to me after exten-

---

LAUREN F. PFISTER, Professor, Department of Religion and Philosophy Humanities, Hong Kong Baptist University; currently Visiting Professor, Institut für Religionswissenschaft, Universität Bern. Specialities: Qing Dynasty philosophy, Confucian–Christian dialogue, cross-cultural hermeneutics. E-mail: feileren@hkbu.edu.hk

sive research in relevant materials in both English and Chinese literature: the need for us who are traditional Chinese philosophers to engage directly and thoroughly the sphere of technological problems and philosophy of technology when addressing problems of environmental ethics. I not only show why this is a critical philosophical issue, but also make a small constructive suggestion to initiate some response. The final two sections move more directly into descriptive ethics, involving a number of practical responses to obvious problems experienced in Hong Kong and China. In this regard, I believe it is important for those interested and involved in contemporary expressions of traditional Chinese philosophical schools to consider the notable lack of practical responsiveness to many major issues related to environmentally sensitive living prior to 2005, and the continuing need to discuss practical problems of relevant implementation. This is because these are matters which pervade not just the lifeworlds of Chinese citizens in general, but also those where our circles of Chinese philosophers in Mainland China as well as in "cultural China" live and teach.

I. Obvious Absences: Chinese Philosophers and Contemporary Environmental Ethics

Though literature on environmental ethics and related fields such as the philosophy of technology have grown into a large corpus of published materials in Anglophone and Chinese worlds during the last forty years, it is remarkable to note how very few Chinese persons, authors, and advocates are identifiable as significant within their circles and collected writings.[2] A major challenge to this pattern occurred when a whole issue of the *Journal of Chinese Philosophy* in March 2005 was devoted to the general theme of environmental ethics. Still, my own impression is that there are troubling factors which make it difficult to identify among ancient, past, and contemporary Chinese philosophers suitable exponents and exemplars for environmental and ecological ethicists. One of the major figures prompting recent developments in environmental ethics, who has invited and prompted discussions of Chinese philosophical texts and themes, J. Baird Callicott, has explicitly sought to address these issues within Chinese and other Asian texts in a way which brings "the natural environment within the purview of ethics" while "keep[ing] human well-being and the human social fabric in sharp moral focus." Admittedly, and Callicott is one of the first to underscore the point, those who do not take up a Neo-Kantian approach to these matters may pursue a form of "deep ecology" or a non-anthropocentric form of ecological ethics that undermines the balance Callicott prefers to maintain.[3]

In 2005 some new alternatives were discussed including discussions of relational, process, and reconstructionist accounts of environmental ethics appealing to Ruist ("Confucian") and Daoist classical precedents,[4] followed by an attempt to present a new synthetic theoretical grounding as a contribution to the contemporary ethical discussion by Professor Chung-ying Cheng.[5] Most of these tried to offer a balanced form of ethical reflection including human, non-human, and more general natural realms in the environing world, but not all with equal success. Notably, a more strong classical Daoist expression of a non-anthropocentric environmental ethics was also articulately presented by Sandra Wawrytko,[6] suggesting just how little consensus there is among current traditional Chinese philosophers in the field. Some others like Wawrytko who advocate non-anthropocentric versions of environmental ethics quite strictly employ ancient Daoist texts and themes to promote their environmental visions, while Callicott and those like him mentioned previously prefer to employ suggestive themes in a varied mixture of Ruist, Daoist, other Asian and native American Indian teachings as parts of a larger ethical scheme balancing environments and humans in ways which do not privilege environment over humans (and other living beings), and so do not become more or less misanthropic.[7]

When one reviews contemporary discussions of environmental and ecological ethics, the general impression is that this area of philosophical study is largely unrepresented in traditional Chinese philosophical circles, even in spite of some notable exceptions. This under-representation should not only become a matter of academic concern among philosophers, but also appear to be quite ironic given the fact of the obvious recent rise since 2004 or so of public awareness in the People's Republic of China (PRC) about environmental problems. Put more directly, in spite of the fact that public interest and even judicial action within the PRC has manifestly become more environmentally self-conscious, most traditional Chinese philosophers rarely address any of the related issues in their own writings.[8] Most of those who actually do write articles about these matters appeal to categories drawn from Marxist traditions and "the laws of natural dialectics" (*ziran biannzhengfa*), yet very few of these persons address the relationship between traditional teachings (*jiao*) and major themes in environmental or ecological ethics.[9] That a few Chinese books in the PRC have appeared during the last five years directly addressing the role traditional teachings may play in relation to these themes is encouraging, but the issues they address, following precedents from cultural China where some more substantial works are also available, still lack a thorough engagement with concerns addressed by natural scientists and philosophers of techno-science. We will discuss the significance of these shortcomings a little later.

Another general angle we can consider regarding the obvious lack of engagement with major trends in these spheres can be drawn from those in Chinese and Anglophone worlds promoting "ecological ethics" (*shengtai lunli*). For example, during the period from 2002 to 2005 members of the Union of Concerned Scientists presented a blistering set of critiques of Bjørn Lomborg's book, *The Skeptical Environmentalist* (2001), challenging its sanguinely optimistic assessment of macro-environmental factors, producing within a year after Lomborg's book was published a number of critical articles in major scientific journals including *Science*, *Nature*, and *Scientific American*.[10] This interesting and wide-ranging debate within international scientific circles has received no basic or sustained response within any Chinese philosophical publications that I have found, suggesting that many are either unaware of or uninterested in these matters, even if they are interested in ecological or environmental ethics. It is this kind of situation which provokes me to consider a number of more self-critical and reflective questions.

II. A Few Puzzling Problems: Questions about What We are not Questioning

In my reading of articles and books related to environmental and ecological ethics, there are times I sit back with genuine puzzlement, wondering why certain themes are not addressed. Sometimes these problems arise in my own mind, I suspect, because there are conflicts between various values which are not thoroughly or consistently worked out among various ethicists; other times, certain claims made in articles and books prompt me to doubt their validity, or are directly challenged by other authors who have already recognized these shortcomings. Happily, some substantial and suggestively creative positions were put forward in 2005 by a group of Chinese philosophers representing primarily Ruist and Daoist philosophies, as already mentioned, but as of yet there is no consensus among them about how to resolve these major problems. Here I intend only to list a few very basic problems which I will not address further, but believe they are significant enough to at least mention at the outset.

Why is it that many Chinese philosophers representing traditional schools of thought generally advocate as a primary value within their environmental ethics the fundamental "promotion of life"? This approach to the question actually camouflages a real diversity regarding the hierarchy of beings among traditional Chinese schools. Most ancient Ruist scholars clearly gave preferences to human beings, even though Master Meng (Mengzi) also spoke of "caring for animals" as part of the extension of human compassion.[11] Master Xun (Xunzi) was particularly adamant in placing the human social network in opposition to a distinctively "unhuman" natural order.[12] In contrast to these more or less anthropocentric visions, Ruist scholars of the Song and Ming Dynasties expressed a more sensitive appreciation for living things in their natural settings, even to the point of projecting some basic attitudes about an organismic relationship between humans and "the myriad things."[13] These later Ruist scholars had already absorbed a significant amount of Daoist interest in the larger natural order.[14] This kind of emphasis on a non-anthropocentric worldview was particularly noticeable in the works of the earliest Daoist philosophers (the *Daodejing* and the *Zhuangzi*), but then developed into a strong empirically oriented search for elements to form an immortal elixir or pill that required careful observation of many aspects and entities in the natural environment (such as in the work of the Wei-Jin period Daoist scholar, Ge Hong).[15]

Responding to a very different account of the environment was the Japanese Buddhist monk, Dōgen (Dao Yuan), whose teachings have attracted the environmental philosopher, Arne Naess, because of its decentering of human experience in the larger context of an environing natural whole.[16] Nevertheless, it is how traditional Chinese philosophers unravel their understanding of "promoting life" that interests us here, and so the diversity of accounts among them—especially as they consider the interrelationships and values of humans, sentient beings, and the environing world—stands in contrast to any simplistic claim that there is a singular "Chinese" view of the matter.[17]

A broader vision of "life," such as that found in Daoist traditions and some Buddhist writings, would manifestly challenge a basic value inherent in quite a number of traditional ethical systems that promote anthropocentric visions of life. Many ethicists understand these alternative worldviews to entail a serious reconsideration of the very nature of ethics itself. They argue that if we reconceive our ethics so that the hierarchy of values they support are not inherently anthropocentric, another basic outlook on "life," and particularly on "human life," would clearly emerge. It is very much in this light that Callicott in 1987 offered a challenging call to encourage "students of Eastern thought [and so here we would highlight Chinese philosophical options] to contribute in a most welcome[d] and important way to the literature of environmental ethics" (Callicot 1987, 128). Some initial responses in English-language books have occurred in the subsequent two decades in Ruist, Daoist, and Buddhist realms, regularly as a joint effort of concerned scholars, but their influence on non-Chinese circles of environmental ethicists and scientists interested in these areas is yet to be seen. Yet what remains awkward, especially for those who read through Chinese language accounts of contemporary environmental ethics which represent the traditional "three teachings," is that there is still much that is significant in the broader contemporary debates in environmental ethics to be addressed.

So, for example, why is it that Chinese environmental ethicists do not assert a reevaluation of our normal vision of life in the light of the natural or systematic role of death in ecological systems? Certainly the *Daodejing* and *Zhuangzi*, whether they are considered to promote "environmentalist thinking" or not,[18] are less bound up with the progressive promotion of anthropocentric forms of life, and the *Zhuangzi* in particular playfully downplays the "normal" human fixation on the "evil" of death. There is also already in the *Analects* of Master Kong ("Confucius") a deep sense of awe for the heavenly decree (*tianming*) that determines the fate of human beings. This attitude has been cited by some late twentieth century new Ruists as an instance of a humanistically oriented spirituality, while among the followers of Wang Yangming's teachings in the sixteenth and seventeenth centuries, there was a profoundly existential concern about the reality of personal death. Whether it ends up promoting what we could now recognize as a new framework for environmental ethics is still debatable.[19]

Similarly, ecologists often argue that the diversity of the biosphere will be better maintained by non-interference in the life-and-death struggles of individual beings. Does not the *Yijing* suggest—in a fashion not unlike the darker voices of Ecclesiastes and Buddhist meditations which seek to empty any attachment to the fear of death—that there will be times of decline and death as well as times for advance and living?[20] Is this one of the alternative *Dao* in Chinese philosophical teachings, which illustrates a contrasting view of life between Ruist and Daoist or Chinese Buddhist traditions?

While the question of the "nature of Nature" has been raised quite early on by Chinese philosophers, particularly but not exclusively by those with a Daoist inclination,[21] there has not been a subsequent engagement with the reflective discussions by neo-Kantian and theistic ethicists who have begun to question the complexities and the relatively modern history of the development of an environing concept of "Nature" in recent years.[22] While Chinese philosophers have often advocated the interrelatedness between humans, sentient beings, the environing lifeworld, and the universe at large, there has not always been a concentrated effort to unpack *both* the ontological *and* epistemological problems inherent in "Nature" itself. While some in other contexts are using these kind of reflections to talk about the "end of

Nature" due to its more inherent conceptual difficulties bound up with a human-other dialectic, many Anglophone accounts of Daoist and Ruist ("Confucian") environmental metaphysics continue to use the term "Nature" as if it is not in itself problematic. Precisely in this context one finds it problematic to have such different accounts of the character of *tian* as "Heaven," or "Nature" itself, or included in "Nature" as "heaven and earth" (*tiandi*), while other writers focus on what is "spontaneous" or "natural" (*ziran*), as if these concepts would not also have to address issues in a post-industrialized transformation of the natural order.[23]

In particular, some opt for what Tu Weiming has promoted on the basis of readings in Gabriel Marcel as the Chinese adoption of an "anthropocosmic vision," which promotes an "organismic" view of the universe and humans' part within it. Here again, whether this particular version of the "human-Nature" connection is "the" Chinese understanding leaves one in puzzlement, since Daoist and Chinese Buddhist alternatives do not always adopt this approach, even in their interpretation of the *Zhongyong*, which Tu employs as his major canonical text.[24] Notably, accounts written in 2005 by Ruiping Fan, Hourdequin and Wong, and Chung-ying Chung—all of whom adopt basic Ruist positions of different sorts—specifically challenge a simplistic reading of any anthropocentric vision.

Another question which I find intriguingly difficult to unravel is one addressed with great care and illustrative power by Callicott in an article seeking to assert the need for a unified moral account of environmental ethics in opposition to a pluralistic moral model which has been promoted by Peter Wenz.[25] Callicott argues that a pluralistic ethical model, while employing different evaluative systems for different ranges of sentient and non-sentient beings, ultimately leads to a conflict of values that threatens to produce moral confusion or unresponsive despair. My own rational inclinations are to agree with Callicott, but my ethical attempts at practicing various matters related to different realms of ethics attune me to the significance of moral pluralist arguments. Unfortunately, for my rational inclinations, I find that the diversity of positions presented as Ruist, Daoist, and Chinese Buddhist approaches to environmental ethics only reinforces this sense of the reality of the plurality of approaches and the moral problematic inherent in pluralistic approaches.

A more pragmatic approach that accepts this diversity of worldviews for the sake of coordinating a positive environmental sensitivity is promoted by Andrew Light.[26] More recently, Professor Chung-ying Cheng has made a valiant effort to synthesize various views, as mentioned previously; his method of thinking "both integratively and pluralistically" is put forward in order to move toward "a unity which solves our common and separate problems better" (Cheng 2005, 347–48). This manifestly goes beyond Light's environmental pragmatism by readdressing a method seeking a theoretically synthetic and comprehensive unity, but requires more thorough consideration and testing by others in order to achieve wide recognition by environmental ethicists in general.

While these puzzlements trouble me as matters for which I continue to seek some basic clarification and more methodological rigor, there are several other problems that provoke me even more poignantly because of their absence in any traditionally oriented account of Chinese environmental or ecological ethics. This involves the manifest absence of any sophisticated account of technology and techno-science within contemporary accounts of Chinese environmental ethics, an issue which is too often camouflaged under the rhetoric of the assuredly "natural" and "uncomplicated" relationship between humans and an environing Nature.

III. CURIOUS OVERSIGHT? TECHNO-SCIENCE, POLLUTION, AND CHINESE TEACHINGS

Many of the most startling and ethically demanding problems arise due to the pervasive extent of pollution, so that Carl McDaniel refers to the "uncomfortable truth" that "the current scale and character of human activities are decreasing the planet's life-support capacity both in known and in unanticipated ways" (McDaniel 2005, 216).[27] My concern, however, is that we Chinese philosophers actually need to take note of several other dimensions of these claims. First, most of these "human activities" are directly linked to technological innovations and the environing influences of techno-science—whether rooted in cars, buses, and transportation technologies or dealing with the production and dispersion of the multitude of modern commodities.[28] Following this, the current environmental and ecological state of our lifeworlds is one where a crisis is immanent, if it has not already fallen upon us. No Chinese scholar needs to be reminded that the majority of the most polluted cities in Asia—clogged by dirty air, stale and trashy water, streets and lands cluttered by discarded waste products, many being biologically undegradable—are in Mainland China.[29] That this degradation has been a conscious element of the Maoist ideology has also been carefully revealed and boldly evaluated in Judith Shapiro's volume, *Mao's War against Nature*.[30]

This being a publicly agreed upon fact, why is it that so very few traditional Chinese philosophers do not discuss the problems of pollution when dealing with environmental and ecological ethical problems?[31] Furthermore, why is there almost no mention, let alone sustained discussion, of the nature and impact of the technological systems and techno-sciences which are complicit in these encroaching environmental and ecological problems? These shortcomings risk leaving a strongly negative impression on those outside the general fields of traditional Chinese philosophy. In effect, it suggests that many efforts devoted to environmental and ecological ethics made by scholars representing these Chinese traditional teachings are essentially anachronous and therefore irrelevant to the actual and concrete conditions of our international macro-environmental crisis. One can hardly help but wince at the stinging rebuke made against two volumes exploring Buddhist and Confucian approaches to ecology by a conscientious but frustrated environmental ethicist in 2000 when he starkly stated:

> [A] pervasive problem in both volumes is the lack of critical reflection on key terms relating to ecology and the environments . . . there is an increasingly diverse range of literature on environmental topics, both in the sciences and in humanities disciplines, and the authors appear to be mostly unaware of the growing terminological sophistication in this area. . . . There is a general lack of sophistication and insufficient attention to methodological problems.[32]

This critical assessment can now be countered at least in part by some seminal efforts since 2000, especially in the March 2005 issue of the *Journal of Chinese Philosophy*. Unfortunately, however, I sense there is still a dramatic need to address matters related to the status of technology, its systems and values, and the roles they have played and continue to play in the twentieth and twenty-first centuries.[33] For example, Professor Chung-ying Cheng ended his very reflective essay "On the Environmental Ethics of the *Tao* and *Ch'i*" with the following comments:

> [Hu]man[s] must recognize that there are visible and invisible elements of nature, and that there are many concentric circles of *ch'i* [*qi*] structures which all can act and react on the well-being of man. Man has to incorporate his understanding of the interpenetration among things in his technological exploration of nature. This is essential for making technology not only humanized, but naturalized as well. . . . In becoming creative, following the *Tao* [*Dao*] will help insure that man's research and invention do not issue from a desire to dominate or result in a will to control. Many things that men have done in history have been a waste of life and energy. This can be avoided by following the creative spontaneity of the *Tao*.[34]

Though this has been stated twenty years ago, it was only in 2005 that some attention to technological concerns were expressed in English literature on environmental ethics by traditional Chinese philosophers, while this is still lacking in Chinese literature in these areas explored by their representatives. Rather than elaborate on other problems related to the effective explanations of the *Tao* and *Ch'i* into hermeneutically accessible ideas for those outside the realm of Chinese philosophy, I will focus on the assumptions still regularly embedded in statements which essentially overlook the ontic status of technology and the deconstructive or even "unnatural" characteristics of techno-scientific systems and some of their tendentious innovations. Can "technology" be "humanized" and "naturalized"? Is there a "natural *dao*" of technology? If so, why has something so "natural" gone so wrong at times? If not, what has made it not so? In speaking about technology are we considering certain machines or, more expansively, larger physical systems created by humans, or do they refer to the extensions of humans' desires to dominate and control?

Furthermore, if all of Nature consists of visible and invisible *qi* ("ch'i"), and noting that *qi* can be both universal and concrete in its conceptual coverage, what kind of *qi* constitutes technological machines or technological systems? Are they just as "natural" as other kinds of things in our lifeworlds? Or do they constitute something other, another form of life that is neither natural or human(e)? If so, how would this be clarified and elaborated in a *qi*-based account of our lifeworlds? In the vast majority of accounts of environmental ethics by traditional Chinese philosophers, even to the present day, I have yet to find a single writing that notes and explores the subtlety of these questions regarding the interrelational ontic intrusions of technologies and technological systems into human experiences and environmental problems. Most often they are subsumed under the rubric of "the natural" in a way that is in fact strikingly unnatural and highly questionable.

Though these questions may be new to Chinese philosophers who approach environmental ethics from the resources of traditional Chinese teachings, they are not at all new to Chinese Marxist philosophers or the other philosophers on whom they rely, both foreign Marxist philosophers and those dealing with philosophy of technology as well as environmental ethics. The "non-neutrality" of technology is a theoretical position developed at great length by Habermas and others, and has only recently (2003) been directly addressed within one philosophically inclined article. Here I myself take a particular theoretical stand, one directly influenced by the formative work of the French intellectual, Jacques Ellul, and those who rely on his insights.[35] To approach a philosophical understanding of technology, we must not merely deal with various kinds of machines or even interlinking systems of machines, but realize the techno-scientific approach to life has produced what Ellul refers to as an alternative "environment." The values inherent in technological systems—seeking the quickest, cheapest, and most effective ways to advance themselves—are those which create an environing techno-world mediating all that we experience.

Technology is an artificial environment which sustains our current way of life, mediates almost everything we do in acting as living things, and is so intimate to our assumptions about living that it at times even threatens our very existence. Those who like Larry Hickman present us with an understanding of technology which deals only with mechanical elements and their physical systems, whether driven by the Deweyian pragmatism Hickman adopts, as in his book, *Philosophical Tools for Technological Culture*,[36] or a more naïve attitude about technology as mere "objects" within our natural environment, have not yet penetrated into the heart of the metaphysical and ethical issues which press us to deal with environmental ethics. Precisely for these kinds of reasons, Steven Vogel talks coherently about thinking ethically "after the end of Nature," because we rarely have any direct contact with natural environments, especially for those who live in large and sophisticated cities. Even what we may purposefully seek to know about "wilderness" is mediated by our transportation to those places in airplanes and automobiles, wearing "appropriate" clothing made elsewhere which protects us from the different climate and physical challenges of trekking on unpaved paths, taking up accommodations in comfortable inns and hotels, and the touristy attitudes we take in slipping in and out of the wild, seeing what is new and even beautiful to us. By all these technologically provided means we actually never have to live within these places as a true "environment" in the Ellulian sense of the term. So too, Andrew Light speaks about making urban environments "environmentally sound," but within his sophisticated pragmatic approach to environmental problems, one wonders if his vision of environmentally sound places is determined more by our technological environment (in Ellulian terms) than by other possible standards (though he clearly appeals to worldviews informed by a number of Christian and Buddhist positions as well as by process philosophy).[37]

Similar questions can also be raised to challenge the more sophisticated accounts found in the March 2005 issue of the *Journal of Chinese Philosophy*, for none of the philosophers there clearly and categorically distinguish technological systems from human(e) and/or natural forms of existence. Technologies, technological systems, and their self-sustaining values are either considered to be human products completely under "our control," or placed within the scope of "natural environment" without any sense that there has been an epochal change in technological intrusions into both human and natural realms.

Exactly what kind of traditional Chinese terminology might be used to explain and interact with this more sophisticated account of the technological environment remains a puzzle to me. An environing *qi* as described previously by Professor Cheng seems to overlook the inherent techno-alterity of the technological environment; the concreteness in an instrumental *qi*, as developed in Wang Fuzhi's more material-oriented and *Yijing* informed philosophy, may be useful, but I sense that it still may not be sufficient in providing an adequate account of the inhumane values inherent in technological systems. Connected to this particular problem of explaining environmental ethics in appropriate ways is another question which has plagued my mind as I have read through relevant literature.

Many of the current writers in traditional Chinese philosophy who address issues in this area are concerned with good reason to promote a new metaphysical and moral account of the relationship of humans to "Nature," however it is conceived. In this process, I sense that there is an overemphasis on the spatial and environing scales of our life-worlds or environments, but far less coherent and direct discussion about the historical and temporal dimensions in the development of environmental ethics as a problem and a discipline.[38] Have we lost a sense of the unprecedented historical nature of the environmental and ecological problems because we have overemphasized our perceived metaphysical advantages in giving an account of the relationship between humans and "Nature"? Have we lost sight of the time periods, timing, and temporal progressions through which environmental pollution increases its accumulative harmfulness, due to our habits of thinking with more spatial, metaphysical, and naturalistic orientations?

In this light we should consider another pressing problem of philosophical importance related to these kinds of inquiries. While some major Chinese philosophers have made some initial forays into the area of environmental and ecological ethics, they continue to adopt older Chinese categories for natural phenomena (especially *qi* rendered as "vital energy," "material energy," "stuff," and "psychophysical stuff") which baffle non-Chinese and non-philosophical readers. By not attempting to provide adequate empirical references to these concepts for readers steeped in techno-scientific terminology and a technological value system, Chinese writings about these traditional categories are very vulnerable to principled neglect.[39] This in fact has been the general fate of the vast majority of materials written about environmental and ecological ethics by contemporary Chinese philosophers representing traditional teachings until 2005; once published, they have been treated as unusual specimens for reading, almost like the contemporary interest developed in reading about paleontological discoveries about extinct dinosaurs. Will we simply allow this to continue?

While it is important to note at this point the relative paucity of traditional Chinese philosophical discussions which engage the otherwise relatively well-developed literature in both Chinese and Anglophone worlds addressing directly or indirectly environmental ethics—a situation recently corrected to some degree by the full issue of the *Journal of Chinese Philosophy* devoted to this theme in March 2005—we should not avoid facing up to various kinds of rather embarrassing academic ironies that appear as a result. For example, Northeastern University in China has been a major center for studies in the philosophy of technology. It hosted a two-week-long international conference focusing on this theme in July and August 2004, the tenth in a series of similar conferences which commenced in 1985. Among the 120 persons involved in the conference were some well-known international participants: the noted American phenomenologist of techno-science from the State University of New York, Don Ihde, the Canadian radical philosopher from Simon Frazer University, Andrew Feenberg, as well as several Japanese scholars among others. Writings by Ihde and Feenberg appear regularly in collections devoted to the philosophy of technology, and both have published important major works in the field.[40]

If we accept as true to the case that technological systems are an intimate part of the matrix which produce polluted environments, that they are not "naturally" present in our environing worlds, and intrude in ways that can be destructive of whole environments, we must take up these interpretive challenges. Knowing that there have been discussions about these technologies and some of their problems in conferences held in the PRC for over twenty years, we are driven to ask ourselves: Why are other Chinese philosophers, especially those working as advocates in traditional schools of contemporary Chinese philosophy, not addressing these matters in greater depth?

IV. Possibilities of Creative Collaboration in Environmental Ethics

Due to the unprecedented scale of Chinese polluted landscapes and the pressing realities of the deterioration of the quality of life in most major cities within Mainland China, I sense that it is high time to consider collaborations that will help those of us engaged in studies of the traditional streams of Chinese philosophy to overcome the current obstacles inherent in our past and present approaches to environmental and ecological ethics. As most of us would understand, there has been a lack of political will reinforced in many dimensions of PRC life, one which has rarely been enfranchised by more engaged forms of legal political activity, and so there seem to be fairly monumental problems of taking up calls for changes in public policies there. Fortunately, as mentioned above, there are apparent changes in this political mindscape. How much can informed Chinese philosophers and those involved in environmental ethics become engaged with shaping government policies related to practical and legal conditions to reorient the general lack of environmental care in the cities and countryside of the PRC? According to Koon-Kwai Wong in 2005, in spite of the emergence of "Green Nongovernment Organizations (NGOs)" in Mainland China in recent years, there has not been much impact felt at the level of government policy changes, in spite of a few notable cases which have begun to receive media coverage in 2006.[41] In Hong Kong we have an Ombudsman that is a governmentally assigned mediator for matters of this sort, where informed citizens have been able to both voice their concerns and begin to influence policies when they lobby legislative representatives about these matters. How much this is feasible, and in what manners this could be done in other parts of the PRC, should be concretely discussed.

Furthermore, there is a growing corpus of discussions about environmental and ecological issues among natural scientists, engineers, and social scientists that begs to be addressed in a more sophisticated ethical manner. Could not an international working group involving noted Chinese ethicists and recognized members of Chinese scientific communities, as well as philosophers of technology and social scientists, be created in order to work out formulations for a viable "environmental ethics with Chinese characteristics"? How could legal initiatives now permitting "Green NGOs" be integrated into local, provincial, and national programs? A good number of the authorized religious groups in Mainland China have also made more or less clear statements about their own religious convictions regarding environmental and ecological concerns, and so they too could be consulted and collaborations worked out.

It would seem appropriate and important to overcome the stigma of trying to assert a "truly Chinese" philosophical approach for environmental ethics and so simply avoid interaction and constructive dialogues over ethical norms and normative practices that should be encouraged and adopted among the various spheres of representative intellectuals in all these groups. Some synthetic and cooperative trends of this sort have already appeared in 2005, where process philosophy and Daoism, bioregionalism and theological environmental concerns have been reflected in Ruist discussions. Some straightforward evaluations of environmentally destructive practices have been theoretically and pragmatically addressed at several different levels of discourse. Once more, would it not be wise for appropriate representatives among contemporary Chinese philosophers working in the traditional schools to coordinate groups of these kind of concerned PRC citizens, helping them to formulate appropriate ways to identify commonly agreed upon norms and a practical program of livable principles which member groups would encourage and realize?[42]

One of my deepest concerns is that there appears to be a manifest lack of moral will on the part of many Chinese philosophers to take up environmental and ecological ethics *and* to live them out in their own personal patterns of life, not to mention making these matters of teaching and imitable models for students and others. Once again, I can note that I have found some rare and hopeful exceptions in recent works by Hourdequin and Wong (2005) and Professor Chung-ying Cheng (2005). Yet in previous years I have wondered, following Antonio Cua's recent ethical reflections on "moral failure" in the *Mengzi*, whether we as Chinese philosophers should have a fundamental "lack of will" to be involved, or a "lack of a sense of moral priority or importance" because of conflicting values, or a basic lack of understanding due to being uninformed technologically and scientifically and so lacking an "appreciation of the nature of the current situation."[43] Though some positive examples to the contrary do now exist in 2007, they are still so few that one is driven to ask some very provoking and practical questions. So in the following I will raise a number of issues of personal and communal practice, believing that such concrete discussions will encourage us all to become philosophically engaged citizens of our various countries, especially for those of us living in the PRC.

V. Practical Provocations and/or Provocations to Practical Environmental Care

If philosophy involves practice, and various traditional Chinese philosophies strongly assert that knowledge and action should be intimately related, I want to ask what those of us who live and serve our communities as Chinese philosophers in our different realms are actually doing to work out responses to the numerous kinds of environmental problems which have to be faced. Certainly, some will rightly point out that the Chinese government and many of its citizens have accepted a one-child policy precisely because of the pragmatic problem of overpopulation and its environmental impact. Though this has remained controversial from various perspectives, the fact is that this policy has addressed one of the two most basic issues which "deep ecology" regularly asserts is fundamentally important in addressing environmental problems: overpopulation and overconsumption. These and the other massive problems related to Chinese polluted landscapes certainly do need to be addressed in governmental policy; in fact, the story of environmental management in the PRC is full of its own snags and obstacles, and is addressed in various volumes published through the Chinese Association for the Protection of the Environment in Beijing. It is important to note that a number of articles that propose "environmentally sound" solutions suggest that one of the strategies is to move away from more democratic and capitalistic forms of lifestyle toward a more restrictive form of political polity in order to deal with these problems.[44] There is a manifest and constant tension here between political freedoms and civic responsibilities that remains a trenchant hindrance to many other possible scenarios for addressing environmental problems. I take it as philosophically significant to address these matters also at personal and familial levels, extending them ultimately into village, town, and city levels.[45]

Water course ways are not only naturally polluted by the force of river flows which ravage topsoils during flooding seasons, but also dramatically affected by casual dumping of sewage, and the leakage of fertilizers and insecticides into streams and rivers. Water shortages—matters of water supply for growing populations particularly in mega-urbs, suburbs, and sizable exurbs both in China and elsewhere—are becoming a matter of regular concern. What are we doing to recycle the more or less limited resources of water for various purposes? Is there a system of using water for multiple purposes, such as taking bath water and rinse water and using it also for watering the garden? Though these are obviously piecemeal approaches to bigger problems, they are significant ways at personal and familial levels to help reduce water consumption and prudent measures to discover a new conservationist approach to water usage.

Air pollution is a matter of increased concern in all major Chinese cities as well as those overseas. What have we done personally and familiarly to respond to these issues? Have we chosen to make use of forms of transportation that do not pollute the environment, even though they are not so efficient? (I am thinking of riding bicycles and driving sun-battery-driven automobiles rather than employing fossil fuel burning motorbikes, motorcycles, automobiles, or buses.) How many of us or our families have self-consciously chosen to walk or ride bicycles rather than drive cars when pursuing local chores?[46] Yet I must say in all honesty that the level of consistency I and my family have achieved on these matters, mostly due to becoming accustomed to transportation conveniences and sometimes being overwhelmed by certain urgencies, has not always been as strong as I would prefer it to be.[47]

How many of our Chinese philosophers and their families protect themselves from the pervasively polluted cityscapes, especially the polluted air, of their university towns? I myself began wearing a pollution mask both in Hong Kong and in Mainland China in the early 1990s, and have found it all the more necessary in the subsequent years. At times it appears awkward, and other times (especially on hotter days) it is not so comfortable; convincing family members to take up this self-protection is also not always easy to do. Nevertheless, the greater the necessity became apparent, the easier it was to change our habits.

Sometimes philosophical concerns move those of us in the professional academy to focus on some very uncomfortable facts, and so I have written here as candidly and carefully as I can about these perplexities, questions, and doubts about how much contemporary Chinese philosophers who work in traditional schools of Ruist, Daoist, and Chinese Buddhist traditions engage environmental and ecological ethics not only as a theoretical matter, but also as a plan for personal, familial, social, and perhaps even political action. If this awkward attempt to struggle with these issues encourages practical engagement of some sort mentioned above, I will rejoice (my celebrations being muffled behind my antipollution mask).

HONG KONG BAPTIST UNIVERSITY
Hong Kong, China

UNIVERSITÄT BERN
Bern, Switzerland

Endnotes

1. I have learned from Jing Haifeng that the phrase "cultural China" was first employed by Charles Fu (Fu Weixun) in order to address practical ways to overcome cross-strait tensions between Taiwan and Mainland China in the 1980s, although Tu Weiming adopted the phrase to refer to non-Chinese scholars of China who are engaged with reflecting on and representing Chinese worlds in significant ways to non-Chinese audiences. Professor Chung-ying Cheng tells me that he also spoke using this same phrase in conversation with journalists in 1979 or so. It is in this latter sense that I use the term.

2. I have found about ten articles devoted to relevant Chinese sources and themes in the journal, *Environmental Ethics*, during its twenty-five years of quarterly publication. The neglect and silence on issues reflecting Chinese themes is even more pronounced in (purportedly) comprehensive anthologies and volumes of environmental ethics published in English. My review of the most recently published volumes on environmental ethics in Beijing's Tsinghua University Press confirmed this general impression: Though technical and scientific discussions of environmental problems were in abundance, none of the recent volumes referred to any discussion of these matters which invoked Ruist ("Confucian"), Daoist, or Buddhist categories of thought.

3. For the quotation and discussion of alternative theories of environmental ethics, see J. Baird Callicott, "The Case against Moral Pluralism," in *Environmental Ethics*, 3rd ed., ed. Andrew Light and Holmes Rolston III (Oxford: Blackwell Publishing, 2003), 203–19, at 203–4. Reference will be made later to this text as (Callicott, 2003), followed by a page number.

4. As found in the following articles: Marion Hourdequin and David B. Wong, "A Relational Approach to Environmental Ethics," *Journal of Chinese Philosophy* 32, no. 1 (2005): 19–33; Alan Fox, "Process Ecology and the 'Ideal' Dao," *Journal of Chinese Philosophy* 32, no. 1 (2005): 47–57; and Ruiping Fan, "A Reconstructionist Confucian Account of Environmentalism: Toward a Human Sagely Dominion over Nature," *Journal of Chinese Philosophy* 32, no. 1 (2005): 105–22.

5. Chung-ying Cheng, "Approaches to Environmental Ethics Reconsidered," *Journal of Chinese Philosophy* 32, no. 2 (2005): 343–48.

6. Sandra A. Wawrytko, "The Viability (*Dao*) and Virtuosity (*De*) of Daoist Ecology: Reversion (*Fu*) as Renewal," *Journal of Chinese Philosophy* 32, no. 1 (2005): 89–103.

7. Callicott draws from a variety of Indian and East Asian teachings in, "Conceptual Resources for Environmental Ethics in Asian Traditions of Thought: A Propaedeutic," *Philosophy East and West* 37, no. 2 (1987): 115–30. He wrote this essay as a constructive and critical response to some of his earlier claims in "Asian Traditions as a Conceptual Resource for Environmental Ethics," *Environmental Ethics* 8, no. 4 (1986): 300–315. Hourdequin and Wong in "A Relational Approach to Environmental Ethics" refer also to two Native American Indian traditions in their discussion.

8. See indications of these developments in Koon-Kwai Wong, "The Greening of the Chinese Mind: Environmentalism with Chinese Characteristics," *Asia-Pacific Review* 12, no. 2 (2005): 39–57; Craig Simons, "Getting Help from the People: Environmental Activists are having an Impact," *Newsweek*, February 14, 2005, 28–29; and Tilman Wörtz, Florian Hanig, and Lu Guang, "China: Der Schwartze Reise" [China: The Black Trip], *GEO: Das Neue Bild der Erde* [*GEO: The New Picture of the Earth*] 11 (2007): 110–138.

9. In my personal research experience, searches using computer search engines in Hong Kong and Melbourne revealed that the vast majority of articles in journal literature from 1994 and the first part of 2005 that deal with "environmental protection" (*huanjing baohu*) were written by natural scientists and engineers who address localized problems in particular sectors of the environment. When I added the selective term "ethics" (*lunli*) to these searches, the field was reduced from over 1,700 items to just seven articles.

10. The final chapter of Carl N. McDaniel's book, *Wisdom for a Livable Planet* [sic] (San Antonio, TX: Trinity University Press, 2005), presents a thorough discussion of this dialectically charged situation (esp. at 220–28, 257–59). McDaniel's book boldly addresses various themes in environmental and ecological ethics, but notably does not include a single Asian or Chinese among its list of imitable persons. Reference will be made later to this text as (McDaniel, 2005), followed by a page number.

11. See Ruiping Fan, "A Reconstructionist Confucian Account of Environmentalism," who also supports an explicit monotheistic Ruist worldview based on a special reading of the *Xici* commentary to the *Yijing*, but then essentially reduces environmental ethics to a specific culturally anthropocentric set of values.

12. Hourdequin and Wong in "A Relational Approach to Environmental Ethics" support a reading of the *Xunzi*, however, that may suggest a more relational basis for environmental ethics, that is, a mutually engaging connection between humans and various levels of environing contexts. This resembles in their minds the work pursued by the bioregionalism movement.

13. See, for example, the recent discussions on ecological concern that have emerged from a Ruist–Christian dialogue on the subject and which focus on key figures such as Zhang Zai, Cheng Hao, and Wang Yangming. Consult Lai Pun-chiu and Lin Hongxing, eds., *Ru Ye Duihua yu Shengtai Guanhuai* [*Confucian–Christian Dialogue and Ecological Concern*] (Beijing: Religious Culture Press, 2006), 180–282.

14. Intriguingly, Ruiping Fan ("A Reconstructionist Confucian Account of Environmentalism") sees these Song Ruist scholars from his reconstructionist point of view as

distorting their tradition with Daoist cosmology, and so losing their original Ruist cosmic worldview, rather than enriching their thoughts synthetically.

15. A highly problematic English rendering of Ge Hong's work was produced by James Ware in the 1960s, but still one can find within its pages sections devoted to natural observations, and proto-scientific hypotheses about the natures of various things. Consult James R. Ware, trans., *Alchemy, Medicine, Religion in the China of A.D. 320: The Nei P'ien of Ko Hung (Pao p'u tzu)* (Cambridge: MIT Press, 1966). With regard to the twenty-first-century classical Daoist readings of environmental ethics, Wawrytko's article ("Viability (*Dao*) and Virtuosity (*De*) of Daoist Ecology") is in principle non-interventionist, while Fox ("Process Ecology and the 'Ideal' Dao") offers a process philosophical reading involving infinite numbers of necessarily conflicting *daos*, and so is explicitly pluralist in his metaphysics while not completely against intervention.

16. This emphasis by Naess is mentioned as one of three major sources for ecological thinking in Andrew Light, "The Case for a Practical Pluralism," in *Environmental Ethics*, ed. Andrew Light and Holmes Rolston III (Oxford: Blackwell Publishing, 2003), 239. Light also points out that others have disagreed with Naess, including Deane Curtin, in "A State of Mind Like Water: Ecosophy T and the Buddhist Traditions," *Inquiry* 39, no. 2 (1996): 239–84.

17. Professor Chung-ying Cheng's ("Approaches to Environmental Ethics Reconsidered") synthetic effort to draw both "earthly" and "heavenly" approaches together, seeking to bridge anthropocentric and non-anthropocentric environmental accounts by means of vantage points including aesthetic, contemplative, and integrative principles in order to overcome "merely postmodern" and "simply pluralistic" accounts of environmental ethics, indicates just how difficult it will be to bring such diversified perspectives into an attractive, justified, and dynamic theoretical position. No consensus exists yet among traditional Chinese philosophers about how such a unified vision for environmental ethics might be achieved. Reference will be made later to this text as (Cheng, 2005), followed by a page number.

18. The question of whether these early Daoist texts should be read as a form of "naturalism" was raised by R. P. Peerenboom in his intriguing article, "Beyond Naturalism: A Reconstruction of Daoist Environmental Ethics," *Environmental Ethics* 13, no. 1 (1991): 3–22. More recently, Paul Goldin has argued for a claim which is a corollary to this problem in "Why Daoism Is Not Environmentalism," *Journal of Chinese Philosophy* 32, no. 1 (2005): 75–87. Supporting the opposite position are Wawrytko ("Viability (*Dao*) and Virtuosity (*De*) of Daoist Ecology") and Fox ("Process Ecology and the 'Ideal' Dao").

19. So, for example, some of the essays in the two-volume set edited by Tu Wei-ming and Mary Evelyn Tucker, *Confucian Spirituality: Volume I* and *Confucian Spirituality: Volume II* (New York: Crossroads Publishing, 2003 and 2004, respectively) reflect on humans' existential condition, but the nature of *tian* itself (which could be rendered as "heaven" or "Nature," depending on the context and intention of the author), remains a basic ambivalence that is not always held consistently by New Ruist advocates. Late Ming developed a manifest and existential concern for issues of life and death. For example, see the essay by Peng Guoxiang entitled "Yangming Xuezhe de Shengsi Guanqie [The Intense Concern about Life and Death among Followers of Wang Yangming]," *Zhexue Pinglun [Philosophical Inquiry]* 4 (2006): 171–88. (I would like to thank my student, Chan Hau-lung, who brought this article to my attention.) Ruiping Fan ("A Reconstructionist Confucian Account of Environmentalism") only addresses ritual awareness of death among humans, but has nothing to say about the dying of other sentient beings of even cultural and natural systems. One senses a greater concern for these areas in Hourdequin and Wong, "A Relational Approach to Environmental Ethics" and Chung-ying Cheng, "Approaches to Environmental Ethics Reconsidered." In this sense, there is a wider range of perspectives about these issues within Ruist traditions, especially when viewed from a historical perspective, than is normally admitted by some Chinese Ruist scholars.

20. For this reason, Ruiping Fan's ("A Reconstructionist Confucian Account of Environmentalism") optimistic reading of "civil society" and its positive virtues through the

Xici commentary to the *Yijing*, which explicitly mentions war in its comments, leads to a less realistic and acceptable interpretation of these matters.

21. This question was apparently first highlighted in the relevant literature by Po-Keung Ip ("Taoism and the Foundations of Environmental Ethics," *Environmental Ethics* 5, no. 4 [1983]: 335–43) and then was addressed more directly in an article a few years later by Roger T. Ames in "Taoism and the Nature of Nature," *Environmental Ethics* 8, no. 4 (1986): 317–50.

22. These include Bill McKibben, *The End of Nature* (New York: Anchor Books, 1989); and more recently Steven Vogel, "Environmental Philosophy after the End of Nature," *Environmental Ethics* 24, no. 1 (2002): 23–40. Most recently this theme has been worked out with much insight and thoroughness in Gerhold K. Becker's article, "Je suis le grand tout: Respect for Nature in the Age of Environmental Responsibility," presented in an international symposium on "Environmental Ethics: An Inter-religious Dialogue" held at Hong Kong Baptist University on June 9–10, 2005. This article will appear in a book edited by Ip King-tak entitled *Environmental Ethics: International Perspectives* to be published by Rudopi in Amsterdam in either 2007 or 2008.

23. Here I am thinking in particular of the dilemma of the "tragedy of the commons," a metaphor initially coined by the biologist Garrett Hardin, which has prompted many environmentalists to adopt this terminology to refer to ecological crises and to consider what actually constitutes the "commons" (see Garrett Hardin, "The Tragedy of the Commons," *Science* 162 [1968]: 1243–48). John Vandermeer offers a nuanced understanding of the "commons" as involving "externalities" within systems of production which are not normally maintained or paid for by market economy-oriented businesses. Consult John Vandermeer, "Tragedy of the Commons: The Meaning of the Metaphor," *Science and Society* 60, no. 3 (1996): 290–306. When this question about the "nature of Nature" is put even more poignantly, we should ask whether Nature, environment, and world are denoting the same or different concepts, and whether they coincide with *tian* and/or *tiandi* in various texts. This ambiguity in the basic denotation of these reference terms brings significant problems at times for Hourdequin and Wong ("A Relational Approach to Environmental Ethics"), and seriously threatens the coherence of Fan's thesis ("A Reconstructionist Confucian Account of Environmentalism").

24. Professor Tu has written several articles promoting this anthropocosmic vision in relationship to environmental ethics in Mary Evelyn Tucker and John Berthrong, eds., *Confucianism and Ecology: The Interrelation of Heaven, Earth, and Humans* (Cambridge: Harvard University Press, 1998). In the edited work he shared with Mary Evelyn Tucker on *Confucian Spirituality: Volume Two*; he ends the second volume with a spirited attempt to show that there is a central "ecological turn" within major ideas promoted in the writings of Contemporary New Ruists. Nevertheless, the ambivalences in the meaning of "Heaven" (*tian*) promoted within varying Ruist texts—which include conceptualizations alternating between a supreme deity, a major element within a cosmic whole, and Nature (or the cosmos) itself—suggest that Tu's ecological reading of this major concept may be misguided.

25. Consult J. Baird Callicott, "The Case against Moral Pluralism," in *Environmental Ethics*, ed. Andrew Light and Holmes Rolston III (Oxford: Blackwell Publishing, 2003), 203–19. The position he takes to task is found in Peter S. Wenz's *Environmental Justice* (Albany: State University of New York Press, 1988).

26. Andrew Light, "The Case for a Practical Pluralism," in *Environmental Ethics*, ed. Andrew Light and Holmes Rolston III (Oxford: Blackwell Publishing, 2003), 229–47.

27. The epochal shift in environmental problems is still not always recognized or accepted by traditional Chinese philosophers. Wawrytko ("Viability (*Dao*) and Virtuosity (*De*) of Daoist Ecology"), Fox ("Process Ecology and the 'Ideal' Dao"), and Fan ("A Reconstructionist Confucian Account of Environmentalism") all tend to downplay or overlook the historical fact of the unprecedented level of environmental problems, while Hourdequin and Wong ("A Relational Approach to Environmental Ethics") and Chung-ying Cheng ("Approaches to Environmental Ethics Reconsidered") candidly note the critical and macro-environmental nature of our current and future ethical problems.

28. By February 2007 there has been confirmation by an international group of scientists supported by the United Nations Framework Convention on Climate Change, that the vast majority of greenhouse gases affecting well-attested climactic changes are known to have been the result of human activities. See their website for details: http://unfccc.int/2860.php. While Professor Chung-ying Cheng ("Approaches to Environmental Ethics Reconsidered"), Hourdequin and Wong ("A Relational Approach to Environmental Ethics"), and Wawrytko ("Viability (*Dao*) and Virtuosity (*De*) of Daoist Ecology") all make great strides in addressing various aspects of pollution and concrete questions of environmental destruction and sustainability, others in the March 2005 issue of the *Journal of Chinese Philosophy* tend to sidestep the issues in ways to be discussed below.

29. Though government policies in Mainland China have permitted the emergence of environmentally active nongovernmental organizations, there are restrictions and political sensitivities that have prevented these new movements from becoming very influential in public and political life. Among those mentioned as key figures in this new area of civic society within Mainland China, one does not find the name of a single Chinese philosopher, not to mention an advocate of one of the three traditional teachings emphasized here. See cogent accounts of these matters in Koon-Kwai Wong's article, "Greening of the Chinese Mind," and Wörtz et al.'s "China: Der Schwartze Reise."

30. Judith Shapiro, *Mao's War against Nature: Politics and the Environment in Revolutionary China* (Cambridge: Cambridge University Press, 2001).

31. This oversight is remarkable, and yet is regularly left unaddressed in numerous essays and books dealing with humans and the natural (*ziran*). But here Chinese philosophers writing in English are just as culpable as those writing in Chinese. One major example in a recent major work is the volume edited by Tucker and Berthrong, specifically entitled *Confucianism and Ecology*. In this book of over 350 pages, the problems of pollution are mentioned on only five pages, and so are hardly discussed in a context where ecological problems are regularly created by these polluting technologies. So far the most sustained discussions of some of these devastating issues are found in Chung-ying Cheng, "Approaches to Environmental Ethics Reconsidered," as well as in Hourdequin and Wong, "A Relational Approach to Environmental Ethics."

32. C. John Powers, review of two volumes: Mary Evelyn Tucker and Duncan Ryūken Williams, eds., *Buddhism and Ecology: The Interconnection of Dharma and Deeds* (Cambridge: Harvard University Press, 1997); and Tucker and Berthrong, *Confucianism and Ecology*. The review appears in *Environmental Ethics* 22, no. 3 (2000): 207–10.

33. The most recent text I have been able to find that offered some hope was the Chinese volume edited by Lai Pun-chiu and Lin Hongxing, *Confucian–Christian Dialogue and Ecological Concern*, but once again there was no direct account of the scientific and technological dimensions of our environmental crises within the whole book.

34. Chung-ying Cheng, "On the Environmental Ethics of the Tao and the Ch'i," *Environmental Ethics* 8, no. 4 (1986): 351–70, at 369.

35. Ellul's seminal works in this area are a three-volume set produced over a period of thirty years. These are translated into English as Jacques Ellul, *The Technological Society*, trans. John Wilkinson (New York: Vintage Books, 1967); Jacques Ellul, *The Technological System*, trans. Joachim Neugroschel (New York: Continuum Publishing, 1980); and Jacques Ellul, *The Technological Bluff*, trans. Geoffrey W. Bromiley (Grand Rapids: William B. Eerdmanns Publishing, 1990).

36. Larry A. Hickman, *Philosophical Tools for Technological Culture: Putting Pragmatism to Work* (Bloomington: Indiana University Press, 2001).

37. See discussions of Light's positions in http://www.terrain.org/essays/13/light.htm. Refer also to Andrew Light and Eric Katz, eds., *Environmental Pragmatism* (London and New York: Routledge, 1996); and Eric Katz, Andrew Light, and David Rothenberg, eds., *Beneath the Surface* (Cambridge: Massachusetts Institute of Technology, 2000).

38. So, as mentioned earlier, there are still a good number of traditional Chinese philosophers writing about environmental ethics who downplay or overlook the epochal significance of the current macro-environmental crises that are now considered undesirable by the vast majority of natural scientists.

39. So even in books which suggest that there might be some important discussions of this sort, the actual content is disappointing in its avoidance of the actual technological dimensions of macroscopic environmental pollution. This is the case in J. Baird Callicott and Roger T. Ames, eds., *Nature in Asian Traditions of Thought* (Delhi: Sru Satguru Publications, 1991); as well as in Peter D. Hershock, Marietta Stephaniants, and Roger T. Ames, eds., *Technology and Cultural Values* (Honolulu: University of Hawai'i Press, 2003). Though the latter volume manifestly recognizes that this general problem exists, there is no sustained presentation of how contemporary Ruist, Daoist, and Buddhist philosophers would address specific technological problems.

40. See, for example, Ihde's contributions to the phenomenology of technological units, systems, and their influence on lifeworlds in his contributions to Robert C. Scharff and Val Dusek, eds., *Philosophy of Technology: The Technological Condition—An Anthology* (Malden: Blackwell Publishing, 2003); and David Kaplan, ed., *Readings in the Philosophy of Technology* (London: Rowman & Littlefield Publishers, 2004). Consult also Andrew Feenberg's incisive account of technology which is responsive to the wider ranges of Marxist and post-Marxian critiques of technology in *Transforming Technology: A Critical Theory Revisited* (Oxford: Oxford University Press, 2001).

41. Consult Koon-kwai Wong, "Greening of the Chinese Mind."

42. Here the assumptions of a democratically based form of political life also need to be qualified and challenged, depending on the national and transnational contexts involved. Especially in the case of the PRC, which has not yet adopted any major democratic political mechanisms into its normal governmental principles at levels of policy making, this assumption leads to unrealistic assessments. This is true even in spite of the more open political context of Hong Kong and Macau, and so the sobering assessments of Koon-kwai Wong ("Greening of the Chinese Mind") need to be carefully considered.

43. These selective quotations come from a set of six possible scenarios set up by Antonio Cua in "*Xin* and Moral Failure: Notes on an Aspect of Mencius' Moral Psychology," in *Mencius: Contexts and Interpretations*, ed. Alan K. L. Chan (Honolulu: University of Hawai'i Press, 2002), 126–50, at 131–32, 134–39, 142–43.

44. See, for example, McDaniel, *Wisdom for a Livable Planet*, 216–28; Stephen Gardiner, "The Real Tragedy of the Commons," *Philosophy and Public Affairs* 30, no. 4 (2002): 387–416; and Alfred Endres, "Increasing Environmental Awareness to Protect the Global Commons—A Curmudgeon's View," *Kyklos* 50 (1997): 3–27.

45. I am grateful to be able to note that in his essay of June 2005 Professor Chung-ying Cheng also addressed many of the following practical concerns. This was a fact I was not aware of when I wrote this article, and learned about only later.

46. For an ethical consideration of these matters in a North American context, see Julia Meaton and David Morrice, "The Ethics and Politics of Private Automobile Use," *Environmental Ethics* 18, no. 1 (1996): 39–54.

47. These comments have stimulated an email dialogue between the editor of this volume, Karen Lai, and myself about our familial ways of adjusting our levels of comfort within urban settings where it is more or less normal to drive automobiles. Though in Hong Kong the vast majority of people are able to use public transport, and it is both efficient and environmentally friendly in form, I still find the calculus for determining when we would use our car, how long we would endure high levels of humidity rather than turn on the air conditioner, particularly when we are with guests, is a pattern that tends to support the more sophisticated account of "the tragedy of the commons" described by Vandemeer (as found in endnote 23 above).

CHINESE GLOSSARY

Chan Hau-lung	陳孝龍	Dao	道
Cheng Hao	程 顥	*Daodejing*	《道德經》
Chung-ying Cheng	成中英	Dao Yuan	道元

Fan Ruiping	范瑞平	tian	天
Fu Weixun	傅偉勳	tiandi	天地
Ge Hong	葛 洪	tianming	天命
huanjing baohu	環境保護	tian ren heyi	天人合一
Ip King-tak	葉敬德	waidan	外丹
jiao	教	Wang Fuzhi	王夫之
Jing Haifeng	景海峰	Wang Yangming	王陽明
Kong Fuzi	孔夫子	Wei-Jin	魏晉
Koon-Kwai Wong	黃觀貴	wenhua zhongguo	文化中國
Lai Pun-chiu	賴品超	Xici	繫辭
Lin Hongxing	林宏星	*Xunzi*	《荀子》
lunli	倫理	"Yangming Xuezhe de Shengsi	
Mengzi	孟子	Guanqie"	
Mengzi	《孟子》	"陽明學者的生死關切"	
Ming	明	*Yijing*	《易經》
Peng Guoxiang	彭國祥	Zhang Zai	張載
qi (vital energy)	氣	*Zhexue Pinglun*	《哲學評論》
qi (instrument)	器	*Zhongyong*	《中庸》
Ru Ye Duihua yu Shengtai Guanhuai		*Zhuangzi*	《莊子》
《儒耶對話與生態關懷》		ziran	自然
shengtai lunli	生態倫理	ziran bianzheng fa	自然辯證法
Song	宋		

ANTONIO S. CUA*

VIRTUES OF *JUNZI*

Throughout the *Lunyu*, we find frequent occurrence of certain terms such as *ren* (benevolence, humaneness), *li* (rules of proper conduct, ritual, rites), and *yi* (rightness, righteousness. fittingness), indicating Confucius's ongoing concern with the cultivation of fundamental virtues.[1] The unsystematic character of Confucius's ethical thought in part reflects his emphasis on the concrete and the particular. Confucius made extensive use of the notion of *junzi*, instead of principles, for explaining ethical virtues and instruction. Plausibly, Confucius's notion of *junzi* reflects his concern for flexibility in coping with changing circumstances. In this light, Confucius's ethical thought, unlike that of Mencius (Mengzi) or Xunzi, is best characterized as an ethics of *junzi* or paradigmatic individuals.[2] In this article I present a reconstruction of some principal aspects of Confucius's conception of *junzi*. I shall offer a way for sorting out the virtues in the *Lunyu*, with special emphasis on *ren* and *yi* as key elements in a virtue of flexibility.

At the outset, let us note some different translations of *junzi*: "superior man" (Legge, Chan, Bodde, and Dubs), "gentleman" (Waley, Lau, and Watson), and "noble man or person" (Giles, Fingarette, Schwartz, and de Bary).[3] Since we are examining the concept in detail in this article, I will leave *junzi* untranslated. In any case, for Confucius, as well as Mencius and Xunzi, *junzi* expresses an ideal of a cultivated, ethical character. Although more explanation is needed to avoid misleading interpretations, the various translations of *junzi* may be viewed as valuable attempts to bring forth the translator's own appraisal of the salient features of this ideal of ethical character in a way that will be intelligible to English readers. Thus, we may regard *junzi* as a sort of *emphatic* term that, in context, serves to accentuate certain ethically desirable and commendable virtues (*meide*) or qualities of an ideal person. In short, it refers to his or her ethical excellences. In general, *junzi* is a paradigmatic individual who sets the tone and quality of the life of ordinary moral agents. A *junzi*

ANTONIO S. CUA (1932–2007), Professor Emeritus, School of Philosophy, Catholic University of America, and Co-editor of *Journal of Chinese Philosophy*. Specialties: moral psychology, comparative philosophy, Confucian ethics. c/o Karyn Lai, School of Philosophy, University of New South Wales. E-mail: k.lai@unsw.edu.au
*Professor Antonio S. Cua passed away prior to the editing of this manuscript. Therefore, the Journal may be unable to properly rectify errors in his original manuscript.

is a person who embodies *ren*, *yi*, and *li*. Every person may strive to become a *junzi* in the sense of a guiding paradigmatic individual, rather than a *xiaoren* (small-minded person). There are of course degrees of personal ethical achievement, depending on the situation, character, ability, and opportunity of individual moral agents.

I. BASIC, INTERDEPENDENT AND DEPENDENT VIRTUES: *REN*, *LI*, AND *YI*

Concern with the basic interdependent virtues of *ren*, *yi*, and *li* also involves particular dependent virtues such as filiality (*xiao*), magnanimity (*kuan*), trustworthiness (*xin*), and courage (*yong*). These particular virtues are called dependent virtues in the sense that their ethical significance depends on connection with the basic, interdependent, cardinal virtues (henceforth, cardinals). Dependent virtues are not subordinate or logical derivatives of the basic virtues.[4] The ethical significance of the particular dependent virtues is determined by *ren* and *yi*, since these are criteria of moral virtues.[5] Of course, when *li* is invested with an ennobling function, it entails the presence of *ren* and *yi*.[6] As Chen Daqi maintains, what Confucius meant by *de*, in the sense of excellence or virtue, has to do with the product of the intersection of *ren* and *yi*. Thus, both *ren* and *yi* may be said to be the constituent and foundational elements of *de*.[7]

In order to avoid misunderstanding, let us note that dependent virtues are virtues, as they reflect personal merits, even though their ethical significance is determined by their connection with one or more cardinals. At issue is their ethical significance, not their value status as deserving of praise in appropriate contexts. Furthermore, their value status may be appreciated in the light of their function as specifications of the concrete significance of the cardinals, which are basically abstract general concepts. To borrow Xunzi's distinction, the cardinals, *ren*, *yi*, and *li*, are *gongming* (generic terms), and dependent virtues are *bieming* (specific terms), that is, terms that specify the concrete significance of the cardinals in particular contexts of discourse.[8]

For elaboration, we may appropriate Chen Daqi's distinction between complete or whole virtues (*quande*) and partial virtues (*piande*). Cardinals (*ren*, *yi*, and *li*) are fundamental virtues. They may be said to be *quan* or complete in the sense that their ethical value is intrinsic rather than extrinsic. In this sense, *quande* are complete or whole (*quan*) virtues. Moreover, these cardinals are relevant to all situations of human life as our actions have always effects on others. On the other hand, *piande* or partial virtues are so-called because their ethical significance is limited, not only in their application to circumstances but also insofar as their ethical value depends on connection with the cardinals. Here, again, we may invoke Xunzi's distinction between *dao* as a whole and its various *pian* or aspects. Xunzi is critical of some thinkers, not because they espoused faulty or irrational doctrines, but because they comprehend only partial aspects of the *Dao*. Mozi, for example, rightly appreciates the importance of uniformity, but he fails to attend to the value of diversity; Songzi rightly appreciates the value of having few desires, but he fails to see the value of having many desires.[9] Says Xunzi, "*Dao* embodies constancy, but encompasses all changes. A single corner is insufficient to exhaust its nature."[10]

In the *Lunyu*, we do find some of Confucius's remarks that mention both cardinals and dependent virtues in the same contexts, for example, *ren*, *zhi* (knowledge, wisdom), and *yong* (boldness or courage) in 14.28; *gong* (respectfulness), *zhong* (loyalty), *jing* (reverence), and *yi* in 16.10; *li* and *zhong* in 3.19; *li*, *yi*, and *xin* (trustworthiness) in 13.4 and 15.18. Once it was reported that the Master taught four subjects: *wen* (culture, cultural refinement), *xing* (conduct of life), *zhong*, and *xin* (7.25).

For heuristic purposes, we may regard dependent virtues as belonging to two different clusters. One cluster consists of those that are closely related to one basic, cardinal virtue rather than another. Another cluster consists of "overlapping" dependent virtues in the sense that they seem especially germane to the practice of one or more cardinals. For convenience, let us introduce the distinction between supportive and constitutive virtues. Supportive virtues are virtues that are genial or helpful, though not necessary, to the development of the cardinals such as *ren*, *yi*, and *li*. Constitutive virtues, on the other hand, are those that are both supportive and constitutive of the quality of the cardinals actualized. In general, virtues can be admired and can also inspire ideal achievement when they are viewed as constitutive features of an achieved state of a person. However, detached from the governing guide of moral ideals, virtues are mere objects of praise that may not possess a transforming significance for moral agents.

Again the distinction between supportive and constitutive dependent virtues is not intended as a dichotomy. Depending on the character and temperament, what is merely a supportive trait in one person may be a constitutive virtue for another. *Kuan* (magnanimity, generosity, broadmindedness), for example, may be constitutive for a person of mild temperament, but merely supportive for another who has an inordinate self-confidence in the practice of *ren*. In the discussion below, although on occasion I propose a specific interpretation, the classificatory question is open to alternative approaches. More-over, the distinction is offered in a tentative spirit. Perhaps, on closer analysis, the distinction may have only a practical, not theoretical value, that is, helpful to individual agent's reflection on how best to constitute his or her character, on which dispositions are the most congenial for development in the light of individual temperament and circumstance.

Constitutive virtues are those that are integral parts of the state of *ren* achieved, and thus may be termed "integral virtues." Below I discuss briefly *junzi*'s basic qualities of character as embodying a concern with the Confucian cardinals and some supportive and con-stitutive virtues as a preliminary to dealing with Confucius's idea of the flexibility or adaptability of *junzi*.

II. *Ren* and Dependent Virtues

Ren, in the broad sense, is Confucius's *dao*, his vision of the good, an *ideal theme* of concern for humanity. The term "ideal theme" is an appropriation of the notion of theme familiar in various linguistic contexts. Unlike ideal norms, ideal themes do not provide precepts, rules, directives, or principles for action.[11] They are ideal points of orientation that have an import for committed agents. Such terms as development, clarification, and expansion are thus quite at home in discussing ideal themes, whereas in the case of ideal norms, terms such as application, compliance, and extension are more appropriate.

Ren is like a theme in literary or musical composition, amenable to polymorphous, creative expressions, depending on the committed per-son's interpretation of the significance of the ideal for his or her life. Fundamentally, *ren* is the love of fellow humans (*Lunyu* 12.22), or affectionate concern for the well-being of humanity. Commitment to *ren* involves benevolence, that is, desire to do good to others as well as to "study the good of others."[12] As Confucius says: "The *junzi* helps others to realize their (ethically) praiseworthy qualities (*mei*); he does not help them to realize their bad qualities (*e*). The small man does the opposite" (12.16).[13] Contributory to and constitutive of the real-ization of *ren*, is the development of particular dependent, constitu-tive virtues such as *zhong* and *shu*. *Zhong* and *shu* are perhaps the most important constitutive or integral virtues of *ren*.[14]

Zhong is often translated as "loyalty, devotion," sometimes, "doing one's best."[15] For constructive interpretation, all these renderings may be used for indicating a unified conception if we adopt, say, Josiah Royce's preliminary definition of "loyalty": "The willing and practical and thoroughgoing devotion of a person to a cause."[16] "Thoroughgoing devotion to a cause" implies constancy (*heng*) and doing one's best to realize the cause or object of one's devotion, that is, in doing one's utmost with one's whole heart and mind (*jinxin*) to realize the object of commitment (*jinji*).[17]

As a self-regarding virtue, *zhong* implies a commitment to a self-governing standard for conduct. The object of one's devotion may be another person. For example, when Fan Chi asked about *ren*, Confucius replied: "While at home maintain your respectful attitude (*gong*); in handling affairs, be reverend (*jing*); in dealing with others, be *zhong*" (13.19). The object of *zhong* may be a person in a superior position. Thus, in one sense, to be *zhong* is to be loyal to someone superior in the social, political hierarchy, especially to a ruler (2.20, 3.10, 12.14);[18] for example, "The ruler should employ the services of his subjects in accordance with rites (*li*). A subject should serve his ruler by *zhong*." Notably, *zhong* also occurs in non-hierarchical sense (1.4, 7.23, 13.19, 16.10). When Zigong asked about friendship, Confucius replied: "Advise them in the spirit of *zhong* and tactfully guide them" (12.23). It is important to note that the object of *zhong* is people in general; it is not confined to either one's superior or equal.[19] As a *ren*-dependent virtue, *zhong* is not a blind devotion to persons or matters of concern. Even a ruler's conduct is also subject to criticism by subordinates (e.g., 13.15, 13.23). In Xunzi's words, the standard for great conduct is "to follow the *dao*, rather than the ruler and to follow *yi* rather than the wishes of one's father."[20]

Let us now turn to *shu*, which expresses the idea of consideration of others. Viewed separately or together, *zhong* and *shu* involve reflection and judgment. *Zhong* expresses loyalty to and conscientious regard for the moral standard or the ideal of *ren*, that is, an attitude of sincerity and seriousness in one's commitment to *ren*; *shu* more especially pertains to other-regarding conduct. A commitment to *ren* is a commitment to realizing *ren* in the personal relations between oneself and another. *Shu* may be said to be "the golden rule" that governs the exemplification of the *ren* attitude. Zigong asked, "Is there a single word which can serve as a guide to conduct throughout one's life?" The master said, "It is perhaps the word '*shu*.' Do not impose on others what you yourself do not desire (*yu*)" (15:24).[21]

In other words, to be guided by *shu* is to use "oneself as a measure in gauging the desires of others"—an idea expressed in *Lunyu* 4.30 and 6.15.[22] In both formulations, what is crucial is the notion of *yu* or desire. It is misleading to say that *shu* concerns the nature of desire in the ordinary sense, for it has more to do with the manner of satisfaction than with the nature of occurrent desires. A plausible explication of *shu* thus requires a distinction between occurrent and reflective

desires. Thus, what I desire now may, on reflection, be something I
ought not to desire.

Zhong and *shu* may be said to be a method of reflection on occurrent desires, for assessing their appropriateness in the context of
human relations. In this way, the exercise of *shu* presupposes a capacity of self-reflection and self-evaluation. To pay heed to *shu* is to deal
earnestly with the question: Do I want my present desire to be satisfied as I want other's analogous desires to be satisfied in a way that
comports with *ren*? The wanting here is a reflective desire. Thus, a
deliberate consideration on the character of occurrent desires has
consequences in terms of the moral character of one's acts. *Shu* as
moral regard has a practical import only when the agent has subjected
his occurrent desires to reflective evaluation in the light of *ren*.

Recall that the vision of *ren* or the good is an indeterminate ideal
theme, and as such it is subject to diverse, concrete specifications
within the lives of committed agents. At any given time, a reasonable
agent would make such a specification based on a partial knowledge
of the significance of the holistic vision.[23] The ideal of impartiality
implicit in the notion of *shu*, as opposed to partiality of the knowledge
of the good, serves as a reminder of one's imperfection or incomplete-
ness of ethical knowledge. By construing the negative formulation of
shu ("What I do not desire, I ought not to impose on others"[24]) as a
counsel of modesty and humility, we can appreciate its importance by
attending to a characteristic of reasonable persons.[25] Modesty pertains to the moderation of one's claims or demands upon others. One
ordinary sense of "reasonable" indicates that a reasonable person will
refrain from making excessive or extravagant demands on others.[26]
More importantly, in the light of the vision of *dao* or ideal of the good
human life, we would expect reasonable, committed persons to be
modest in making their demands and requests, because no one possesses the knowledge of all possible, concrete, and appropriate specifications of the significance of the good for individual human life.

Let us consider briefly some other *ren*-dependent virtues. On one
occasion responding to a question about *ren*, Confucius said that a
man of *ren* practices five things: "*Gong* (respectfulness), *kuan* (magnanimity, generosity, open-mindedness), *xin* (trustworthiness, being
true to one's words), *min* (agility, adroitness), and *hui* (beneficence)"
(17.6). I suppose that *kuan* and *hui* are dependent, constitutive virtues
of *ren*, for *ren* is basically expressed in love, or affectionate concern
(*ai*). Similarly, warm-heartedness (*wen*) is also *ren*-dependent, constitutive virtue (1.10). *Ren* as an affectionate concern for others would
also be expressed in loving-kindness (*ci*) (2.20), in some contexts,
would be expressed in *kuan*. *Hui* or beneficence is also an expression
of *ren* concern. *Xin* seems to be another constitutive virtue of *ren*, as

indicated in the pairing of *zhong* and *xin* (1.8, 1.9, 9.21, 15.19). For instance, when Zizhang asked about conduct (*xing*), Confucius replied: "Make *zhong* and *xin* your master guides" (15.6). As *zhong* involves doing one's best on behalf of the object of loyalty, *min* (adroitness or agility) would be a virtue of resourcefulness in handling affairs on behalf of the object of loyalty. While *gong* is a dependent, supportive virtue of *li*, it is also a supportive virtue of *ren* when the spirit of *ren* informs its expression according to *li*. As Confucius remarked: "If a man has no *ren*, what has he to do with *li*" (3.3). Moreover, as involving *rang*, *gong* would be merely supportive as in the case of the agent's refusal to yield (*rang*) to his teacher in the practice of *ren* (15.36). As we shall see, *jing* (reverence) is a constitutive virtue of both *ren* and *li*, since it is an essential attitude required in filial conduct (*xiao*)—a foundation for the practice of *ren* (1.2; 2.7).

At this point let us interpose by briefly attending to *keji* and *yong* as *overlapping*, constitutive virtues of *ren*, *li*, and *yi*. When Yan Yuan asked about *ren*, Confucius said: "To return to the observance of the *li* through self-control (*keji*) constitutes *ren*" (12.1). Elsewhere, Confucius also remarked, "If a man has no concern for *ren*, what has he to do with *li*?" (3.3). These two sayings show the interdependence of *ren* and *li*. Self-control is constitutive of the practice of *ren* as it involves overcoming emotions and desires that may well hamper the *ren*-performance. The *li*, as delimiting the proper boundary for the pursuit of self-satisfaction, are the means for self-control. In the case of *yi*, self-control regarding self-serving desires is indispensable to its exercise. *Yong*, as an aretaic or virtue term, is perhaps best rendered as "courage"—the quality of character that shows itself undaunted in facing danger despite fear or lack of confidence.[27] *Yong* is clearly a dependent virtue of *ren*, for "the *ren* person certainly possesses *yong*, but a *yong* person does not necessarily possess *ren* (14.4). Moreover, the person would even sacrifice his life in order to realize *ren* (15.10). Likewise, *yong* is a dependent virtue of *li*; for its ethical significance depends on its connection with *li*. It is an open question whether *yong* is a constitutive virtue of *li*. Arguably, a person committed to the observance of *li*, in some context, may need *yong* to act in the absence of knowledge of the detail rituals involved. Here the agent may need *yong* in the sense of boldness or audacity, a sense of venture, risking embarrassment or humiliation, or even shame.[28] In the case of *yi*, *yong* is clearly a dependent, constitutive virtue. For example, when Zilu asked: "Does the *junzi* cherish *yong*?" The Master said: "For the *junzi*, it is *yi* that is considered supreme. Possessed of *yong* but devoid of *yi*, a *junzi* will make trouble, but a small man will be a brigand" (17.23). That *Yong* is constitutive of *yi* seems evident in this passage: "To see *yi* (the right thing to do) and leave it undone shows a lack of *yong*" (2.24). At any rate, *yong* requires learning (17.8), knowledge, and judgment, which inform the exercise of *yi*.

III. DEPENDENT VIRTUES OF *LI*

Fundamentally, an action conforming to a ritual requirement of *li* has its ethical significance, because such an action is performed in the light of a concern for *ren*. Without a regard for *ren*, ritual observances would amount to mere formal gestures devoid of moral substance. Notably, in addition to imposing restraint on human behavior, as Xunzi points out, the *li* also support the satisfaction of desires (*geiren zhi qiu*) within the defined boundaries of proper conduct.[29] And when a *junzi*'s compliance with *li* is informed by the spirit of *ren*, *li* has also an *ennobling* quality, exemplifying the *junzi*'s respect for *li* as an ideal, *ren* embedded tradition.[30] This attitude toward *li* signifies also a respect for the reality of the situation, the background, and the context for successful moral performance. The Confucian emphasis on *li* is one justification for the Confucian homage to the concrete. If we accept this stress on *li*, some sort of *convention* for identifying the normative import of action seems an essential element in any moral theory. Granted the importance of ethical convention or tradition, attention to the aesthetic and religious dimensions of *li* will also lead us to an appreciation of valuable facets of human life in different cultures and civilizations.[31]

Perhaps the most important dependent virtues of *Li* are *gong* and *jing*. Both terms pertain to expression of respect for others. For distinguishing *gong* from *jing*, we may say that the former pertains primarily to outward appearance, the latter to one's inner attitude. As Zhu Xi put it: "*Gong*'s principal focus is appearance (*rong*), *jing* on human affairs. *Gong* is seen in outward expression (*wai*), *jing* focuses on what is within (*zhong*)."[32] This explanation is supported by Confucius's remark that among the nine things that occupy *junzi*'s thought is "to think of appearing respectful (*gong*) when it comes to demeanor (*mao si gong*)" and "to think of being reverent when attending to human affairs (*shi si jing*)" (16.10). Differently put, *gong* pertains to one's bearing or deportment. *Jing*, however, pertains to virtuous conduct, more specially to one's inner attitude. The idea is also present in the *Yijing*:

> Being straight means correctness, and being square means *yi* (righteousness). The *junzi* applies *jing* to straighten the internal life (*nei*) and *yi* to square the external life (*wai*). As *jing* and *yi* are established, one's virtue will not be an isolated instance.[33]

Another important *li*-dependent virtue is *rang*, which can be rendered in two different ways: "to decline politely (*tuici*)," and *rang*, as in Mencius's *cirang zhi xin*—the seed of the virtue of *li*—has to do with "yielding" (*Mengzi*, Gong Sun Chou I, 2A:6; trans. Legge, *The Four Books* [1981]: 548–52). In both cases, *rang* may be considered as an example of concern with *gong*. One should yield to others in some circumstances, say, in dealing with one's parents or elders, as one may respectfully decline their request. In either case, as we shall see later, the exercise of reasonable judgment in accordance with *yi* is a crucial determinant.

Perhaps the most prominent dependent and constitutive *li*-dependent virtue is *wen* (culture, cultural refinement). *Wen* is reported to be one of the four subjects of Confucius's teachings (7.25). For Confucius, the *junzi* who is "widely versed in culture but brought back to essentials by the *li* can, I suppose, be relied upon not to turn against what he stood for" (6.27). Although the *li*, viewed in abstraction from performance, is fundamentally a code of formal rules of proper conduct, apart from its connection with *ren*, it has an aesthetic aspect. Learning is for the sake of self-improvement, not for the sake of impressing other people (14.24). Xunzi would add, "The *junzi* uses learning to beautify his own person (*mei qi shen*)."[34] Implicit in the idea of *wen* is the beautification of character in the light of cultural refinement. The idea of *wen*, in the light of the connection of *li* with *ren*, in effect, appertains to the ennobling character of persons. Alternatively, *wen* expresses the ennobling function of *li*.[35] In light of this, the *junzi* is a "beautiful" person, as his life and conduct exemplify the "beauty of virtue" in an eminent way, reminiscent of the common concern with "the beauty of virtue and the deformity of vice" among the British Moralists of the eighteenth century.

As a dependent virtue of *li*, a regard for *wen*, as Xunzi would put it, is "to honor the roots" of human existence.[36] However, exaggerated emphasis on *wen* without regard to *zhi* has dubious ethical value. Confucius said, "When there is a preponderance of [native] substance (*zhi*) over acquired refinement (*wen*), the result will be churlishness. Only a well-balanced admixture of the two do we have a *junzi*" (6.18).

IV. *YI* AS THE VIRTUE OF FLEXIBILITY

The well-balanced admixture of native substance (*zhi*) and cultural refinement (*wen*) does not indicate the ideal, for fundamentally *yi* is the substance (*zhi*) of the ethical life (15.18). *Yi* is the Confucian virtue of flexibility. According to Confucius, the *junzi*, in his dealings with the world, "is not invariably for or against anything." He is on the side of *yi* (4.10). Recall also Confucius's autobiographical remark: "I have no preconceptions about the permissible or impermissible (*wu ke wu buke*)" (18.8). Freedom from predilection, prejudgment, inflexibility, and egotism is said to be characteristic of Confucius.[37] These qualities may also be ascribed to the *junzi*, qualities which are necessary to maintain his freedom of thought and action in advance of encounter with particular problematic situations, although Confucius, perhaps out of modesty, disclaimed being a *junzi* (14.28).[38]

If *yi* is "to square with" the external life of the *junzi*, then its primary function is to deal with matters external to the individuals, seen as demands or requirements that need to be made compatible with their inner life and concern. These external demands may appear in the form of duties imposed by custom or tradition, along with institutional rules and regulations, more generally, demands for compliance with *li* as a set of formal prescriptions for proper behavior. This sense of *yi*, which is functionally equivalent to *li*, is often rendered as "duty." The *Liji*, for example, mentioned ten duties of human relationships (*renyi*), such as "The father's loving-kindness (*fuci*) the son's filial piety (*zixiao*), gentleness on the part of elder brother (*xiongliang*), and obedience (*dishun*) of the younger brother."[39]

The *li*, as a corpus of rules of proper conduct, can be quite complex and burdensome even for the committed person. The vastness of the rules staggers our imagination. A chapter (*Liqi*) in the *Liji* alluded to three hundred "great" or important rules (*dali*) and three thousand rules of lesser importance (*xiaoli*), but points out that "they all lead to the same thing." *Yi*, in the sense of rightness, appropriateness, or fittingness, would be the basis of modification of *li*. Moreover, the relevance of the *li* to the present, particularly exigent situation, is a matter of reasoned judgment based on his sense of appropriateness or *yi* and appreciation of the regulative, supportive, and ennobling functions of *li*.[40] Therefore, the *li* are subject to revision or even elimination.

In sum, concern for *yi* is generally a concern for right conduct, which is deemed fitting or appropriate to a particular situation. However, one problematic area of conduct, to use Xunzi's expression, is our fondness for profit or personal gain (*haoli*). In Confucius's words, "The *junzi* understands what constitutes right conduct (*yi*); the small-minded man understands what is profitable" (4.16). In situations where we are tempted to do what promotes our personal gain, Confucius would counsel that "when you see something that is likely to promote personal gain, you must think of right conduct (*jian de siyi*)" (14.12; 16.10), that is, whether the contemplated, self-serving act is the right thing to do. This contrast between *yi* and self-serving benefit suggests the Confucian distinction between morality and egoism.[41] Perhaps for this reason, *yi* is sometimes translated as "moral" or "morality."

V. Dependent Virtues of *Yi*

Let us consider some of the dependent virtues of *yi* as a virtue of flexibility. The idea of *kuan*, with respect to its cognitive purport, expresses a concern with the "largeness" of mind, with catholicity and neutrality, which are the main supportive and constitutive virtues of *yi*. Earlier, we mentioned *kuan*, as a dependent, constitutive virtue of *ren*; that is, *kuan* expresses magnanimity, generosity, or liberality. For elaborating the complex notion of *kuan* as a constitutive virtue of both *ren* and *yi*, we may appropriate Xunzi's conception of three desirable qualities of participants in argumentation. Xunzi says of the argumentative discourse of the scholars and *junzi*: "With a humane mind (*renxin*) he explains his ideas to others, with a learning mind (*xuexin*) he listens to their words, and with an impartial mind (*gongxin*) he makes his judgment."[42]

A different way of indicating the virtue of *kuan*, in light of Xunzi's remark and his distinction between generic (*gongming*) and specific terms (*bieming*), is to say that *kuan* is a generic term (*gongming*) for a composite virtue, which may be concretely specified in three virtues: humane mind (*renxin*), learning mind (*xuexin*), and impartial mind or fair-mindedness (*gongxin*). In the context of the exercise of *yi*, *renxin* expresses a concern with the harmful effects of one's conduct on others. More especially in speech, *renxin* would counsel the agent to be vigilant (*shen*) in using words that may hurt others' feelings. Says Xunzi, "Hurtful words engender wounds deeper than those inflicted by spears or halberds."[43]

Gongxin, impartiality or fair-mindedness, is a specific virtue of *kuan*, a characteristic of the *junzi*'s neutrality and catholicity. *Xuexin*, the learning mind (for Xunzi, in discourse), is the virtue of receptivity, that is, the ability to listen to others without prepossession or prejudgment. In *Lunyu*, Confucius frequently stresses on the importance of extensive study or learning (*boxue*) and application (6.27, 1.1). As Confucius said, "Learning without thinking is labor lost. Thinking without learning is perilous" (2.15).[44] Another supportive and constitutive virtue of *yi* is *shen*, caution in speech and conduct, which is essential to the exercise of *gongxin* or impartiality, as well as *renxin*. *Gang* or *gangyi* (13.27), resoluteness in commitment to *yi* and the decisiveness in judgment according to *yi*, is also an important supportive and constitutive virtue of *yi* for it is an indispensable prerequisite to its exercise. So also, like *shen*, *gang* is a supportive and constitutive virtue of *ren*.

Perhaps the most important supportive and constitutive virtue of both *ren* and *yi* is *yong* (courage). Confucius said, "The determined scholar and the man of *ren* will not seek to live at the expense of *ren*.

136   ANTONIO S. CUA

They will even sacrifice their lives in order to realize *ren*" (15.10).[45] In connection with *ren, yong* is *the courage to be.* In the context that requires the exercise of *yi, yong* is the *courage to do* the right thing. In sum, *yong* is an overlapping, dependent, constitutive virtue of both *ren* and *yi*.

The foregoing discussion presents a map of the virtues of *junzi,* consisting of cardinal, interdependent virtues such as *ren, li,* and *yi,* and their dependent supportive and/or constitutive virtues. The distinction between interdependent and dependent virtues is a heuristic device for sorting out the virtues. I make no claim as to completeness or to a sharp division of dependent virtues as belonging to one cardinal rather than another, for as I have pointed out, there are overlapping dependent virtues of *ren* and *yi* such as *yong* and *kuan.*

There is a complementary way of grouping the dependent virtues suggested by *Zhongyong,* section 27: honoring moral character (*zun dexing*) and following the path of inquiry and learning (*dao xuewen*), much reminiscent of Aristotle's distinction of virtues of character, and virtues of intelligence in *Nicomachean Ethics.*

Dependent virtues of *ren* and *li* are essentially the virtues of character, and those of *yi,* virtues of intelligence. Notably the virtues of intelligence are complementary to the virtues of character, and they comprise a few virtues not particularly emphasized by Aristotle, but the idea of *phronimous* or man of practical wisdom seems implicit in the idea of the exercise of *yi,* which may be elaborated by Xunzi's conception of *zhilu* or wise and well-informed deliberation, a topic I discussed elsewhere.[46]

For concluding this study of the virtues of *junzi,* let me briefly remark on some problems that call for further exploration.[47] On our map for the virtues of *junzi,* in the distinction between basic, cardinal, interdependent virtues and dependent, supportive/constitutive virtues, it may be said that the unity of virtues is presupposed without argument. This is a difficult issue that deserves extensive discussion. In studying this issue in Xunzi's moral philosophy reported in two articles in the 1980s, I proposed what I called the completion thesis. Concisely stated, this thesis is that *ren, li,* and *yi* are interdependent concepts, for an adequate explication of one must involve the other concept.[48] This thesis pertains to *ideal* unity of virtues, since *ren,* in the broad sense, is an ideal theme. Given the interdependence of these cardinals, the ideality of *ren* will also pervade through the ennobling function of *li* and the exercise of *yi* as exemplified in *renxin* or humane mind. Converting the ideality of the unity of virtues into the actuality of the practice of the virtues is not a theoretical task. In spirit, our thesis on the interdependence of the cardinals is akin to that of J. L. Ackrill and Elizabeth Telfer in their defense of the Aristotelian unity of virtues as an *ideal unity of virtues*, rather than empirical thesis.[49] It is a task for Confucian normative ethicists to inquire into the respects in which our thesis needs to be recast in the light of actual experiences of the conflict of virtues. When such a task is successfully carried out, we may have to revise our thesis into a "limited thesis of the unity of virtues."[50]

Also, for developing an adequate Confucian ethics of virtue, there is the crucial task of elaborating both its theoretical and practical significance, and presently, of dealing with difficult problems attendant to our discussion of *yi* as a virtue of flexibility, for example, such problems as the role or status of ethical rules and principles, and the possible contribution of Confucian ethics as an ethics of character or *junzi* to contemporary virtue ethics, as well as to deontology and consequentialism.

CATHOLIC UNIVERSITY OF AMERICA
Washington, D.C.

Endnotes

An earlier version of this article was presented as the keynote address at the International Conference on Confucianism (Toronto, September 1–2, 2005). I am grateful to Professor Vincent Shen and the organizing committee for providing me this opportunity to present what is one of the main topics of interest in my early years of teaching. After extensive study of concepts of human nature, rituals, reasoning and argumentation, structure of basic Confucian concepts and the unity of knowledge and action in Confucian philosophy, I have returned to Confucius's conception of *junzi*. It seems to me that this conception offers a way to contribute to the recent revival of virtue ethics. More importantly, the conception has inherent import, quite apart from its relevance to current problems and issues in moral philosophy or normative ethics. I am grateful to Karyn Lai and Kim-chong Chong for helpful suggestions in preparing the final version for publication.

1. See Antonio S. Cua, "Reflections on the Structure of Confucian Ethics," *Philosophy East and West* 21, no. 2 (1971): 125–40, incorporated in *Dimensions of Moral Creativity* (University Park: Pennsylvania State University Press, 1978), chap. 4. For an extensive discussion of the conceptual framework of Confucian ethics, see Antonio S. Cua, *Moral Vision and Tradition: Essays in Chinese Ethics* (Washington, DC: Catholic University of America Press, 1998), essay 13.
2. Cua, *Dimensions of Moral Creativity*, chaps. 2–4.
3. James Legge, trans., *The Four Books* (Taiwan: Culture Book Company, 1981); Fung Yu-Lan, *A Short History of Chinese Philosophy*, trans. and ed. Derk Bodde (New York: Macmillan, The Free Press, 1948), 38–48; Homer H. Dubs, trans. with notes, *The Works of Hsuntze* (London: Arthur Probsthian, 1928); Wing-tsit Chan, trans., *A Source Book in Chinese Philosophy* (Princeton: Princeton University Press, 1963); Arthur Waley, trans., *The Analects of Confucius* (New York: The Modern Library, 1938); D. C. Lau, trans., *Confucius: The Analects* (Middlesex: Penguin, 1979); Burton Watson, trans., *Hsün Tzu: Basic Writings* (New York: Columbia University Press, 1963); Lionel Giles, *Sayings of Confucius* (London: John Murray, 1907); Herbert Fingarette, *Confucius: The Secular as Sacred* (New York: Harper and Row, 1972); Benjamin Schwartz, *The World of Thought in Ancient China* (Cambridge: Harvard University Press, 1985); and Wm. Theodore de Bary, *The Trouble with Confucianism* (Cambridge and London: Harvard University Press, 1991).

4. The distinction between basic and dependent virtues is not the distinction between basic and subordinate virtues mistakenly attributed to me by Schoper, citing my earlier article: Antonio S. Cua, "Hsun Tzu and the Unity of Virtues," *Journal of Chinese Philosophy* 14, no. 4 (1987): 381–400. See Jonathan W. Schoper, "Virtues in Xunzi's Thought," in *Virtue, Nature, and Moral Agency in the* Xunzi, ed. T. C. Kline and Philip J. Ivanhoe (Indianapolis: Hackett, 2000), 69–88. For elaboration of the relation between basic, interdependent virtues and dependent virtues, see Cua, *Moral Vision and Tradition*, essay 13.

5. In *Dimensions of Moral Creativity* (51–57, 67–69), I considered *ren* as an internal criterion of morality and *li* as the external criterion. Since the application of *li* as rules of propriety is determined by *yi*, *yi* can also be regarded as an internal criterion, as it is an exercise of judgment concerning the applicability of *li*. Moreover, "just as *jen* (*ren*) cannot be practiced without *li*, or the cultural setting, *jen* cannot be realized without *i* (*yi*), or the judgment of the relevance of *jen* and *li* in concrete situations of moral performance." In *Moral Vision and Tradition*, based on a modification of Chen Daqi's work on *Lunyu*, I discussed the criteria for determining the central or fundamental concepts in the *Lunyu*. See Chen Daqi, *Kongzi Xueshuo* (Taipei: Zhengzhong, 1977).

6. See Antonio S. Cua, "The Concept of *Li* in Confucian Moral Theory," in *Understanding the Chinese Mind: The Philosophical Roots*, ed. Robert E. Allinson (Hong Kong: Oxford University Press, 1989), 209–35. For a more extensive account, see Cua, *Moral Vision and Tradition*, essay 13.

7. Chen Daqi elaborates *ren* and *yi* as constituents of *de*: "The core of *ren* is *ai* (affectionate concern), thus *ai* is the main concern of *ren*. The fundamental nature of *yi* is appropriateness (*yi*), thus appropriateness is the main concern of *yi*. Consider *xin* (trustworthiness or being true to one's words). Because of affectionate concern for people, one will not allow people to be deceived. One's words must be suited to the action, and action must be suited to the words. This is the core of *ren*. In order to abide by fairness (*zhongken*), and for the sake of obtaining good results, one should adhere to *xin* only if such adherence is appropriate and should not adhere to *xin* if such adherence is inappropriate. This is the fundamental nature of *yi*." Chen goes on to distinguish *ren* and *yi* from particular virtues by way of the distinction between complete virtues (*quande*) from partial or incomplete virtues (*piande*). The former are said to be "perfect virtues free from any defects whatsoever. If a virtue has the *ren* element but does not possess the *yi* element, it can only be called a partial virtue" (Chen, *Kongzi Xueshuo*, 230). Chen's distinction is quite different from my distinction between basic interdependent and dependent virtues, for at issue is not completeness or possession of both *ren* and *yi*, but the ethical significance of particular virtues. In other words, in the absence of the connection to *ren* and *yi*, particular virtues may have non-ethical values and may well be commendable from the prudential point of view, provided, of course, they are not exercised contrary to *ren* and *yi*. As I will discuss shortly, Chen's distinction is valuable for elaborating my own.

8. For further discussion, see Antonio S. Cua, *Ethical Argumentation: A Study in Hsun Tzu's Moral Epistemology* (Honolulu: University of Hawai'i Press, 1985), 42–43, passim; and Antonio S. Cua, "The Problem of Conceptual Unity in Hsun Tzu and Li Kou's Solution," *Philosophy East and West* 39, no. 2 (1989): 115–34; incorporated in *Human Nature, Ritual, and History: Studies in Xunzi and Chinese Philosophy* (Washington, DC: Catholic University of America Press, 2005). Note that Chen Daqi employs the same distinction in distinguishing "whole" and "partial virtues."

9. See *Tianlun Pian*, 381. Translations of *Xunzi* are provided by the author unless otherwise stated. Sections of the *Xunzi* and page numbers, as cited in this paper, refer to Li Disheng, *Xunzi jishi* (Taipei: Xuesheng, 1979), which was based on the standard Wang Xianqian's *Xunzi jijie*, 2 vols. (Beijing: Zhonghua shuju, 1988).

10. See *Jiebi Pian*, 478. See also *Tianlun Pian*, 381.

11. For the distinction between ideal norm and ideal theme, see Cua, *Dimensions of Moral Creativity*, chap. 8.

12. See Francis Hutcheson, *An Inquiry Concerning Moral Good and Evil*, 158. This is part II of *An Inquiry into the Original of Our Ideas of Beauty and Virtue; in Two Treatises* (London: J. and J. Knapton, et al., 1729), 158.

13. In this translation, I read *mei* as *meide*, ethically admirable qualities or virtues. All translations of the *Analects* are by the author, unless otherwise stated.

14. The interpretation proposed below is a reconstruction that makes no claim to being faithful to the original text. It draws some materials from two articles: Antonio S. Cua, "Confucian Vision and the Human Community," *Journal of Chinese Philosophy* 11, no. 3 (1984): 226–38; and Antonio S. Cua, "Reasonable Persons and the Good: Reflections on an Aspect of Weiss' Ethical Thought," in *Philosophy of Paul Weiss*, Library of Living Philosophers, ed. Lewis E. Hahn (La Salle: Open Court, 1995), 495–514. Here I discuss *zhong* and *shu* as distinct, supportive, and constitutive virtues of *ren*. This interpretation does not deal with *zhong-shu* as a pair, thus leaving open the interpretative issue. For a brief critical survey of different interpretations of *zhong* and *shu* as a related pair, see David S. Nivison, "*Zhong* and *Shu* (Loyalty, Reciprocity)," in *Encyclopedia of Chinese Philosophy*, ed. A. S. Cua (New York and London: Routledge, 2003), 882–85. See also David S. Nivison, "Golden Rule Arguments in Chinese Moral Philosophy," in *The Ways of Confucianism: Investigations in Chinese Philosophy*, ed. David S. Nivison and Bryan W. Van Norden (La Salle: Open Court, 1996), 59–76.

15. See Lau, *Confucius: The Analects*, Introduction, xv. Note that Confucius occasionally paired *zhong* and *xin* (trustworthiness). *Xin* is also an important dependent virtue. For an informative, historical survey, see Kwong-loi Shun, "*Zhong* and *Xin*," in *Encyclopedia of Chinese Philosophy*, ed. A. S. Cua (New York and London: Routledge, 2003), 885–88.

16. Adopting this definition implies no commitment to Royce's conception of "loyalty to loyalty" as a supreme good. See Josiah Royce, *The Philosophy of Loyalty* (New York: Macmillan, 1920), 16–17.

17. Zhu Xi, *Sishu Jizhu* (Hong Kong: Taipingyang, 1980), 23.

18. Presumably, these passages are partly the basis for Nivison's view that *zhong* is to be construed as "loyalty" as expressing the standard governing the conduct of an inferior to a superior or to an equal.

19. For this reason, Chen Daqi endorses Zhu Xi's interpretation of *zhong* as *jinji*. This interpretation is plausible when we draw attention to its ethical basis in *ren*. See Chen, *Kongzi Xueshuo*, 236–37. See endnote 16 above.

20. *Zidao Pian*, 651.

21. See also 5.12: "Zigong said, 'While I do not wish others to impose on me, I also wish not to impose on others.'" For a similar translation in Modern Chinese, see Mao Zishui, *Lunyu Jinzhu Jinyi* (Taipei: Shangwu, 1977), 248.

22. This is Lau's gloss. Lau continues: "It is interesting to note that when Tzu-kung (Zigong) remarked that if he did not wish others to impose on him neither did he wish to impose on others. Confucius' comment was that this was beyond his ability." See Lau, *Confucius: The Analects*, 135, n. 7.

23. For a discussion of the Confucian notion of reasonableness as contrasted with rationality, see Antonio S. Cua, *The Unity of Knowledge and Action: A Study in Wang Yang-ming's Moral Psychology* (Honolulu: University of Hawai'i Press, 1982), chap. 4; and more generally, Antonio S. Cua, "Ideals and Values: A Study in Rescher's Moral Vision," in *Praxis and Reason: Studies in the Philosophy of Nicholas Rescher*, ed. Robert Almeder (Washington, DC: University Press of America, 1982), 176–208.

24. See *Lunyu* 12.12 and 15:23.

25. See Robert Allinson, "The Confucian Golden Rule: A Negative Formulation," *Journal of Chinese Philosophy* 12, no. 3 (1985): 305–15; and Antonio S. Cua, "Reasonable Persons and the Good: Reflections on an Aspect of Weiss' Ethical Thought," in *Philosophy of Paul Weiss*, Library of Living Philosophers, ed. Lewis E. Hahn (La Salle: Open Court, 1995), 495–514.

26. Kurt Baier, *The Moral Point of View* (Ithaca: Cornell University Press, 1958), 316.

27. Other renderings of *yong* are possible in different contexts, for example, "bravery, boldness, being daring, audacity, fearlessness." One passage (14.28) clearly says that

a *yong* person has no fear (*yongzhe buju*). (See also 9.29.) I leave the translation issue open, since my discussion deals only with the relation of *yong* to *ren*, *li*, and *yi*.

28. For the Confucian conception of shame, see Antonio S. Cua, "Ethical Significance of Shame: Insights of Aristotle and Xunzi," *Philosophy East and West* 53, no 2 (2003): 147–202; incorporated in *Human Nature, Ritual, and History*.

29. *Lilun Pian*, 417.

30. For a discussion of the three functions of *li*, see Cua, "The Concept of *Li* in Confucian Moral Theory." More extensive discussion of *li* and its connection with *ren* and *yi* is given in my *Moral Vision and Tradition*, essay 13.

31. See Antonio S. Cua, "The Ethical and Religious Dimensions of *Li*," *Review of Metaphysics* 55, no. 3 (2002): 501–49; incorporated in *Human Nature, Ritual, and History*. A shorter version of the same title appeared in Weiming Tu and Mary Evelyn Tucker, eds., *Confucian Spirituality*, vol. 1 (New York: Crossroads, 2003), 252–88. For the notion of Confucian ethical tradition, see Cua, *Moral Vision and Tradition*, essay 12.

32. Zhu Xi, *Sishu Jizhu*, 91. Author's translation.

33. *Zhou Yi*. Chan renders *jing* as "seriousness" (*Source Book*, 264). *Jing*, rendered as "reverence" in the sense of "deep respect" for something or someone is a serious, attentive state of mind. This point is consistent with Graham's remark that the word *jing*, as used by the Cheng brothers (Cheng Hao and Cheng Yi), "cannot be translated by 'reverence'"; and Bruce's "seriousness" is utterly inadequate, although accusation can be made against Bruce, it is difficult to find a better alternative. The two aspects of *ching* are interdependent; to collect oneself, be attentive to the person or thing implies that one respects him or takes it seriously; and to be respectful implies that one is collected and attentive. But there is no English word which covers both, and the only course seems to use "reverence" for one and a different word for the other. See A. C. Graham, *Two Chinese Philosophers: Ch'eng Ming-Tao and Ch'eng Yi-ch'uan* (London: Lund Humphries, 1958), 69.

34. *Quanxue Pian*, 19.

35. See endnote 30 above.

36. *Lilun Pian*, 424: "*Guiben zhiwei wen.*"

37. *Lunyu*, 9.4: "There were four things the Master refused to have anything to do with: he refused to entertain conjectures or to insist on certainty; he refused to be inflexible or to be egotistical" (author's translation).

38. The same remark in 9.29. On another occasion, Confucius said, "In the knowledge of letters and the arts, I may perhaps compare myself with other men. But as for the character of a *junzi* who carries out in his personal conduct what he professes—that is something to which I have not yet attained" (7.32).

39. Wang Mengou, *Liji Jinzhu Jinyi*, 2 vols. (Taipei: Shangwu, 1977), 1:301. For a critical discussion of the virtues associated with the five human relationships, see Antonio S. Cua, "*Li* and Moral Justification: A Study in the *Li Chi*," *Philosophy East and West* 33, no. 1 (1983): 1–16; or "Human Relationships and the Virtues," in *Human Nature, Ritual, and History: Studies in Xunzi and Chinese Philosophy* (Washington, DC: Catholic University of America Press, 2005), 63–67.

40. For the notion of *yi* as appropriateness (*yi*), see *Zhongyong*, sec. 20 in Chan, *Source Book*, 104. For this notion of *yi* and its general significance as ruling on the relevance of moral rules to particular circumstances, see Antonio S. Cua, "Concept of Paradigmatic Individuals in the Ethics of Confucius," *Inquiry* 14, no. 1 (1971): 44–45; elaborated in *Dimensions of Moral Creativity*, chaps. 5 and 6. Similar interpretation may be found in Chung-ying Cheng, "*Yi* as a Universal Principle of Specific Application in Confucian Morality," *Philosophy East and West* 22, no. 3 (1972): 269–80; Lau, *Confucius: The Analects*, Introduction, 49–50; and Chen Daqi, *Kongzi Xueshuo*, chap. 3.

41. See Cua, *Dimensions of Moral Creativity*, 67–69.

42. See *Zhengming Pian*, 524.

43. *Rongru Pian*, 55: "*Shangren zhi yan, shenyu maoji.*"

44. Legge's translation of 2.15. For other passages on thinking and learning, see 15.31, 15.32.

45. This is a revised Legge's translation of 15.9.

46. See Antonio S. Cua, "The Possibility of Ethical Knowledge: Reflections on a Theme in the *Hsun Tzu*," in *Epistemological Issues in Ancient Chinese Philosophy*, ed. Hans Lenk and Gregor Paul (Albany: State University of New York Press, 1993), 159–83; incorporated in *Human Nature, Ritual, and History*, essay 6.
47. In my keynote address to the Eleventh Conference of the International Society for Chinese Philosophy held in Taipei in 1999, I mentioned other problems: "What is the role of the developing tradition as the background of Confucian ethics? To what extent can the ideal of *dao* or *ren* be concretely specified in a conceptual framework comprising *ren, li,* and *yi*? How are these fundamental notions to be further shaped to accommodate the evolving normative problems in the ethical life today and tomorrow, problems that are quickly acquiring greater transcultural and global significance? In the context of inter-traditional and/or intercultural ethical conflict, what degree of success can one expect from the employment of my proposed ground rules or transcultural principles of adjudication, such principles as non-prescriptivity or cultural integrity, mutuality, procedural justice, rectification, and reconsideration? (See Cua, *Moral Vision and Tradition*, essay 14.) Perhaps additional or other principles will do a better job in conflict resolution." See Antonio S. Cua, "Problems of Chinese Moral Philosophy," *Journal of Chinese Philosophy* 27, no. 3 (2000): 269–85.
48. See Cua, *Human Nature, Ritual, and History*, essays 4 and 5.
49. Elizabeth Telfer, "The Unity of Moral Virtues in Aristotle's *Nicomachean Ethics*," *Proceedings of the Aristotelian Society* (1989–90): 35–48.
50. See Neera-Kapur Badhwar, "The Limited Unity of Virtue," *Nous* 30, no. 3 (1996): 306–29.

CHINESE GLOSSARY

ai	爱	gongming	共名
boxue	博学	gongxin	公心
Chen Daqi	陈大齐	guiben zhiwei wen	贵本之谓文
Cheng Hao	程颢	haoli	好利
Cheng Yi	程颐	heng	恒
ci	慈	hui	惠
cirang zhi xin	辞让之心	jian de siyi	见得思义
bieming	别名	*Jiebi Pian*	《解蔽篇》
dali	大礼	jiug	敬
dao	道	jinji	盡己
dao xuewen	道问学	jinxin	尽心
de	德	junzi	君子
dishun	弟顺	keji	克己
e	恶	*Kongzi Xueshuo*	《孔子学说》
Fan Chi	樊迟	kuan	宽
fuci	父慈	li	礼
gang	刚	*Liji*	《礼记》
gangyi	刚毅	*Liji Jinzhu Jinyi*	
geiren zhi qiu	给人之求	《礼记今注今譯》	
gong	恭	*Lilun Pian*	《礼论篇》

Liqi	《礼器》	wu ke wu buke	无可无不可
Lunyu	《论语》	xiao	孝
Lunyu Jinzhu Jinyi		xiaoli	小礼
《论语今注今譯》		xiaoren	小人
Mao Zishui	毛子水	xin	信
mei	美	xing	行
meide	美德	xiongliang	兄良
mei qi shen	美其身	xuexin	学心
Mengzi	孟子	Xunzi	荀子
Mengzi	《孟子》	Yan Yuan	颜渊
min	敏	yi (appropriateness)	宜
pian	偏	yi (rightness)	义
piande	偏德	*Yijing*	《易经》
quande	全德	yong	勇
Quanxue Pian	《劝学篇》	yongzhe buju	勇者不惧
rang	让	yu	欲
ren	仁	*Zhengming Pian*	《正名篇》
renxin	人心	zhi (wisdom)	知
renyi	仁义	zhi (native substance)	质
Rongru Pian	《荣辱篇》	zhilü	知虑
shangren zhi yan, shenyu maoji		zhong	忠
傷人之言，深於矛戟		zhongken	中肯
shen	慎	*Zhongyong*	《中庸》
shu	恕	*Zhou Yi*	《周易》
Sishu Jizhu	《四书集注》	*Zidao Pian*	《子道篇》
Songzi (or Song Jian)	宋子, 宋鈃	Zigong	子贡
Tianlun Pian	《天论篇》	Zilu	子路
tuici	推辞	zixiao	子孝
Wang Mengou	王梦鸥	Zizhang	子张
wen (culture)	文	1	
wen (warm heartedness)			
温			

JOURNAL OF CHINESE PHILOSOPHY

The *Journal of Chinese Philosophy* is a peer-reviewed philosophical journal devoted to the study of Chinese Philosophy and Chinese thought in all their phases and stages of development and articulation.

In our view there are three main efforts among recent studies of Chinese philosophy which merit specific mention. First, there is an attempt to make available important philosophical materials (in careful translation) from the history of Chinese philosophy, which constitute a contribution to the scholarly understanding of Chinese philosophy in its original form. Second, there is an attempt to make appropriate interpretations and expositions in Chinese philosophy, which constitute a contribution to the theoretical understanding of Chinese philosophy in its truth claims. Third, there is an attempt to make comparative studies within a Chinese philosophical framework or in relation to schools of thought in the Western tradition, which constitutes a contribution to the critical understanding of Chinese philosophy and its values. All three efforts will be recognized and incorporated in this journal as fundamental ingredients. To better articulate these efforts, we wish to emphasize in this journal employment of critical and rigorous methodology of analysis, organization, and synthesis, for we believe that Chinese philosophy, including those parts which have been labeled mystical, can be intelligently examined, discussed, and communicated. We will thus aim at clear and cogent presentation of ideas, arguments, and conclusions. We will honor creative work in Chinese philosophy—for we ask imagination as well as scholarship in our approach to various aspects and dimensions of Chinese philosophy.

As a summary statement of the intended comprehensive scope of this Journal, we shall mention four major historical periods and five major fields of discipline in Chinese philosophy. The four major historical periods are Classical Chinese Philosophy in Pre-Ch'in and Han Eras, Neo-Taoism and Chinese Buddhism, Chinese Neo-Confucianism, and Modern and Contemporary Chinese Philosophy since the nineteenth century. The five major fields of discipline are Chinese Logic and Scientific Thinking, Chinese Metaphysical Theories, Chinese Moral Philosophy and Philosophy of Religion, Chinese Art Theories and Aesthetics, and Chinese Social and Political Philosophies. We hope that a cross fertilization of these periods and fields will yield a still greater wealth of insight and ideas on nature, life, society, government, and human destiny.

Contributions are now invited in all these periods and fields from all those who take a serious interest in Chinese philosophy and Chinese thought regardless of their orientation. Short and critical reviews are welcome. Special attention will be given to articles dealing with narrow topics with broad significance. In the future, plans will be made for organizing issues on specifically prescribed topics of contemporary interest.

Manuscripts should be typewritten on $8\frac{1}{2}''\times 11''$ bond paper, and articles should be under 20 pages (approximately 8000 words) and book reviews within 6 pages (approximately 2500 words). All texts should be double-spaced. Endnotes (no footnotes) should be placed at the end of the author's text. Two copies of each article or review, and a CD (preferably in Microsoft Word for Windows '95 version or later) are required. Chinese characters are to be transliterated according to the pinyin system. Authors are responsible for the accuracy of all quotations and for supplying complete references. For details regarding the formatting, contact Dr. Linyu Gu via email at linyu@hawaii.edu.

All manuscripts, books for review, and editorial correspondence should be addressed to the editor:

Professor CHUNG-YING CHENG
Editor-in-Chief
Journal of Chinese Philosophy
Department of Philosophy, University of Hawaii
2530 Dole Street, Honolulu, Hawaii 96822, U.S.A.
Telephone: (808) 956-6081
Fax: (808) 956-9228
E-mail: ccheng@hawaii.edu

JOURNAL OF CHINESE PHILOSOPHY

Journal of Chinese Philosophy (ISSN 0301-8121 [print], ISSN 1540-6253 [online]) is published quarterly by Blackwell Publishing, with offices at 350 Main Street, Malden, MA 02148, USA, PO Box 1354 Garsington Road, Oxford, OX4 2DQ, UK, and PO Box 378 Carlton South, 3053 Victoria, Australia. Phone: US (800) 835-6770 or 781-388-8599, UK +44 (0) 1865 778315, Asia +65 6511 8000; Fax: US (781) 388 8232, UK +44 (0) 1865 471775, Asia +61 3 8359 1120; Email: customerservices@blackwellpublishing.com; **Information for Subscribers:** For new orders, renewals, sample copy requests, claims, change of address, and all other subscription correspondence, please contact the Journals Department at your nearest Blackwell office.

Subscription Rates for Volume 34, 2007:

	The Americas†	Rest of World‡
Institutional Premium Rate*	$651	£469
Personal Rate	$85	£69 (€103)

* A Premium Institutional Subscription includes access to full text articles from 1997 to present, where available. Print and online-only rates are also available (see below).

† Customers in Canada should add 7% GST or provide evidence of entitlement to exemption

‡ Customers in the UK should add VAT at 5%; customers in the EU should also add VAT at 5%, or provide a VAT registration number or evidence of entitlement to exemption

For more information about Blackwell Publishing journals, including online access information, terms and conditions, and other pricing options, please visit www.blackwellpublishing.com or contact our customer service department, US (800) 835-6770 or (781) 388-8599, UK +44 (0) 1865 778315, Asia +65 6511 8000.

To purchase back issues before 2000, contact Dr. Linyu Gu at linyu@hawaii.edu. **Back Issues:** Back issues are available from the publisher at the current single issue rate. **Microform:** The journal is available on microfilm. For microfilm service, address inquiries to University Microfilms International, 300 North Zeeb Road, Ann Arbor, MI 48106-1346, USA.

Mailing: Periodicals postage rate is pending at Boston, MA and additional mailing offices. Mailing to rest of world by Singapore Post. Postmaster: Send all address changes to *Journal of Chinese Philosophy*, Blackwell Publishing, Inc., Journals Subscription Department, 350 Main Street, Malden, MA 02148-5020.

Advertising: For information and rates, please visit the journal's website at www.blackwellpublishing.com/jocp, or contact the Academic and Science Advertising Sales Coordinator at journaladsUSA@bos.blackwellpublishing.com; 350 Main Street, Malden, MA 02148; Phone: (781) 388-8532; Fax: (781) 338-8532.

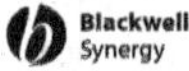

Email Updates: Sign up to receive Blackwell *Synergy* free e-mail alerts with complete *Journal of Chinese Philosophy* tables of contents and quick links to article abstracts from the most current issue. Simply go to www.blackwell-synergy.com, select the journal from the list of journals, and click on "Sign-up" for FREE email table of contents alerts.

Abstracting and Indexing: Arts & Humanities Citation Index, Current Contents, I B Z-Internationale Bibliographie der Geistes- und Sozialwissenschaftlichen Zeitschriftenliteratur, International Bibliography of the Social Sciences, Internationale Bibliographie der Rezensionen Geistes- und Sozialwissenschaftlicher Literatur, M L A International Bibliography of Books and Articles on the Modern Languages and Literatures, Philosopher's Index, Répertoire Bibliographique de la Philosophie, Russian Academy of Sciences Bibliographies, Personal Alert.

Disclaimer: The Publisher and Editors cannot be held responsible for errors or any consequences arising from the use of information contained in this journal; the views and opinions expressed do not necessarily reflect those of the Publisher and Editors, neither does the publication of advertisements constitute any endorsement by the Publisher and Editors of the products advertised.

Printed and bound by CPI Group (UK) Ltd, Croydon, CR0 4YY

07/07/2026

14916218-0004

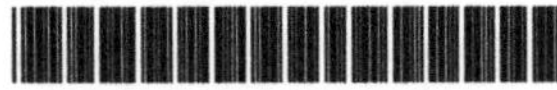